Coping with HEADACHE

Dr DAMIEN ANCIANO

Chambers

© Damien Anciano, 1987

Published by W & R Chambers Ltd Edinburgh

All rights reserved. No part of this publication may be reproduced, stored in a retrieval system, or transmitted, in any form or by any means, electronic, mechanical, photocopying, recording or otherwise, without the prior permission of W & R Chambers Ltd.

Illustrated by Duncan Inglis

British Library Cataloguing in Publication Data

Anciano, Damien
  Coping with headaches.—(Coping with. . .).
  1. Headache—Treatment 2. Self-care, Health
  I. Title
  616'.0472   RC392

ISBN 0-550-20518-7

Typeset by Bookworm Typesetting Ltd, Edinburgh
Printed by Eyre & Spottiswoode Ltd, Thanet Press, Margate

Contents

1. WHO CAN BE HELPED BY THIS BOOK? 1
2. LEARNING ABOUT HEADACHES 14
3. THE MEDICAL APPROACH 30
4. RECORDING YOUR HEADACHES 41
5. LEARNING HOW TO RELAX 52
6. YOUR LIFESTYLE AND YOUR HEADACHES 78
7. DIET, ALLERGIES AND HEADACHES 92
8. ALTERNATIVES 109
USEFUL ADDRESSES 119
FURTHER READING 125

Damien Anciano is a Clinical Psychologist working in a Community Mental Health Team in Colchester. He spent 3 years researching the treatment of problem headaches with relaxation techniques.

In memory of Christine

Acknowledgements

My thanks to Dr Derek Roger and Professor Peter Venables for their assistance in the original research project, and to the Medical Research Council of Great Britain for their financial support. Thanks also to Anna and Stef for help with proof-reading and typing.

1. Who Can be Helped by This Book?

This book is for people who suffer frequent or severe headaches and who would like to learn more about their problem. It is for those people who want to learn ways in which to cope with or reduce their headaches, by changing their diet and using relaxation techniques. The book is aimed at those who suffer one of the two main types of headache, *migraine* and *tension* headache. The self-help treatments described are designed for these headaches. However, those who suffer other types of headache may still benefit. They can learn about the scientific background to headaches, and may indeed be helped by the treatment programme. The truth is that although we know that many sufferers *are* helped, we know very little about who actually benefits from each of these treatments. Try as many different approaches as you can and see which works out best for you.

This chapter will help you identify what kind of headache you suffer from. To do this properly, you may need to record in detail your symptoms as they occur. Memory is notoriously unreliable; all of us tend to remember the worst things about an unpleasant event and forget the less traumatic bits. This chapter will help you decide what kind of headache you suffer from, once you have noted all of the symptoms that go with your headache. And, more importantly, it will also explain when you should seek further help from your doctor.

In Chapter 2 some of the theories about why we get headaches are explained and Chapter 3 describes the medical treatments available from your doctor. Details of how to make a record of your headaches is given in Chapter 4. Chapter 5 explains how relaxation can help headaches and tells you how to relax! How your lifestyle can affect your headaches is considered in Chapter 6 and the next chapter (7) is concerned with the effect of diet on your headaches. Chapter 8, the last chapter, considers alternative medicine and what it has to offer in the control of headaches.

What Kinds of Headache are there?

The vast majority of people who have frequent or severe headaches suffer from one of two kinds. These are *migraine* and *tension* headache. The symptoms that will show you whether you suffer from one of these are discussed later on in this chapter. There are also many other less common types of headache; most of these are due to physical injury or illness and should always be treated by a doctor.

It may seem simple that there are only two types of common headache. All you have to do is note your symptoms and look to see whether your headaches are migraine or tension headaches. However, in reality things are a bit more complicated. There are different kinds of migraine headache, for instance – this means that people who suffer from 'migraine' often have very different symptoms. It also means that the medical treatment may differ according to the type of migraine that you have. The three most common types are called *common* migraine, *classical* migraine, and *cluster* headache. The differences between these are described in the next section on migraine symptoms.

Another complicating factor is that people often suffer *combination* or *mixed* headaches. 'Mixed' means that sometimes you have a migraine headache, and sometimes a tension headache. People can normally tell the difference, but if not then this chapter will help you to do so. 'Combination' headaches are the really awkward ones because these are headaches in which symptoms of both migraine and tension headache exist at the same time. It is not known how often these occur, partly because the symptoms of migraine are so overwhelming that people

Who Can be Helped by This Book

often do not notice the less obvious symptoms. Here again, a detailed record will help. However, deciding exactly which kind of headache you suffer from does not seem to have much bearing on whether or not the treatments described in this book work. This is especially true with relaxation exercises, which seem to help most types of headache. The dietary approach has been scientifically tested mainly with migraine cases, but there seems to be no reason why it cannot be just as effective with tension headaches.

Lastly, there does seem to be quite an overlap between migraine and tension headache. Some people have *all* of the symptoms of migraine, and *none* of the symptoms of tension headache. Others have the reverse. However, many have only one or two symptoms of migraine and maybe some of tension headache. Also, headaches can change over a person's lifetime. They may change at random, so that sometimes they are more like migraines while at others they are more like tension headaches. Or they may gradually change as you get older, one way or the other. Because of this overlap some experts believe that migraine and tension headache are not completely separate clinical problems. They believe that a headache is a headache, and as it gets more severe then more migraine-type symptoms occur. There may be something in this approach; although there are medicines that specifically help migraine or tension headaches, many treatments seem to help both.

The main symptoms that will show you what kind of headache you suffer from are listed in Table 1. Because nothing is black-and-white, the table is just a guide. Remember, keeping a detailed record will help you find out which symptoms you get. You can then look at the table and decide which type of headache yours seems to be.

In the next section the symptoms of migraine are discussed in more detail. You may not have understood all of the terms in Table 1, and there is such a wide variety of symptoms that to put them all into one table would make it too large and confusing. Also, some of the symptoms of migraine can be frightening because they are so strange; if you have some of these then the following section may set your mind at rest. However, if you are at all worried, then *go and see your doctor*. Treatments for *any* kind of headache should always start with medical investigations.

Migraine Symptoms

If there are specific 'trigger' factors; if you have any odd visual or other types of sensation or 'warnings'; or if you are sick during your headache, then it is likely that you suffer from migraine as opposed to tension headache. It may be helpful to describe in more detail these special features of migraine, and how the various types of migraine differ from one another. Cluster headache will be dealt with separately, because in many ways it is a special case, even though it is seen as a type of migraine. Indeed, it is so different that some experts see it as a completely separate kind of headache.

'Triggers' of migraine attacks

Migraines differ from tension headaches in that often there are particular 'triggers' that lead to an attack. They do not always trigger a headache – whether or not they do can depend on how stressed or worn-out you are. Worry, stress and tiredness in themselves are common triggers of both migraine and tension headaches; these are discussed in more detail in the next chapter. In fact, stress is the most commonly reported trigger for both types of headaches. It is worth mentioning here that often a migraine will follow the end of a period of stress while tension headaches tend to occur during the stress. However, the *triggers of migraine are much more specific*. The most common things that may set

Who Can be Helped by This Book

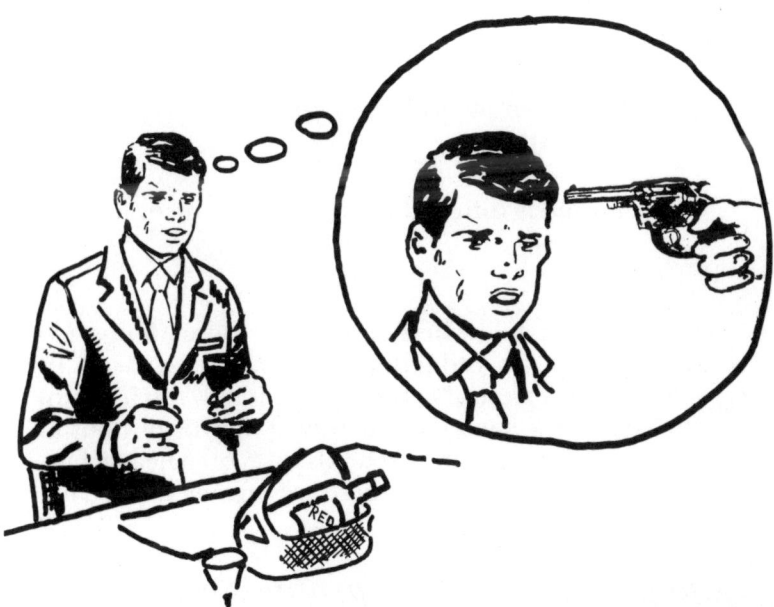

off both classical and common migraines are listed below.

- Excitement
- Menstruation (often the day before your period starts)
- Oral contraceptives (the pill)
- Cigarette smoke or other fumes
- Bright lights or glare
- Noise
- Physical exertion or exercise
- Change in the weather
- Sleep (not enough or oversleeping)

- Hunger

- Alcohol (generally within an hour of having a drink, often red wine)

- Certain foods (often cheese, chocolate or oranges)

- Coffee

How you can tell whether one of these things (or something else) is indeed a trigger is discussed in Chapter 4. The effect of certain foods is also discussed in greater depth in Chapter 7. Anyway, it may be obvious to you that one or more of this list tends to set off a headache – in which case it is possible that these are *migraine* headaches.

Strange sensations or warning signs

Warning signs. In both classical and common migraine, people sometimes report a sense of wellbeing on the day before an attack. They have an ability to think more clearly and to pack many more things into the day than normally. Often, however, these people act a bit irrationally and may ignore the fact that these feelings are a warning that a migraine attack is on its way.

Other people have reported a feeling of mounting tension before a headache. Hunger or reduced appetite can also occur. However, some people report quite bizarre sensations or visual effects that accompany or come before their headaches. This is called the migraine *aura*. If you want to know why the aura happens then Chapter 2 will explain – here some of the sensations that can occur will just be described. If any of these sound similar to your own experience, then you suffer from *classical* migraine attacks. (See Table 1.) If you get no aura but still have the other symptoms of migraine, then you suffer from *common* migraine. Common migraine is just that – probably between five and ten times as common as classical migraine.

		TYPE AND SITE OF PAIN	DAILY PATTERN	COMMON TRIGGERS	RELIEVING FACTORS	SPECIAL FEATURES
M I G R A I N E	CLASSICAL MIGRAINE	Throbbing pain at the front of the head, starting on one side of the head only.	Often on waking and at weekends.	Sometimes none. Alcohol is a common trigger and sometimes particular foods and drinks.	Rest or sleep; a dark room. Certain medications particularly ergotamine (see Ch.3)	Visual effects or other bizzarre sensations. Nausea and/or vomiting. Family history.
	COMMON MIGRAINE	Can be at the forehead, temples or back of the head. A throbbing or stabbing pain; often behind the eye and worse on one side.	Often on waking or late in the day.	Nervous tension, noise, bright lights, periods, certain foods or drinks.	Rest, a dark room, preventative drugs. (see Ch.3)	Nausea and/or vomiting. Family history. Much more common in women, and often linked to the menstrual cycle.
	CLUSTER HEADACHE	At the front of the head and particularly in the eye. Generally on one side of the head. A very severe, stabbing pain.	Occurs at night and like clockwork. Attacks last from 20 minutes to 2 hours.	Sometimes alcohol.	None.	Usually men only, aged between 30 and 50. Bloodshot eyes, tears, blocked or runny nose. Occurs in 'clusters'. (See text).
	TENSION HEADACHE	Tight, pressured pain, often around the whole head, sometimes the neck as well.	Worse towards the end of the day.	Stress, anxiety and nervous tension.	Sometimes tranquilisers. Holidays.	Often other signs of stress or anxiety.

TABLE 1.

People generally have one or the other of these two types of migraine, and do not switch between them.

Changes in vision. Many different kinds can occur in classical migraine. They can involve one or more of the following list:

- Horseshoe or 'C'-shaped patterns
- Flashes of colour
- 'Catherine wheels'
- Zig-zags
- Wavy lines
- Stars
- Spots

These can happen anything from one hour to half a minute before a headache. Some people actually hallucinate, or 'see' things that appear real. For instance, one woman saw skunks with erect tails moving around just before her headaches! In all these cases, however, the person knows that she is seeing things, as opposed to being fooled into believing that it is real. Other people report less dramatic visual symptoms, such as a general blurring of their sight. One person described it 'as if looking through steam or water'.

Other sensations. Some people also suffer temporary numbness or tingling in parts of their body, particularly in the hand or forearm and sometimes the face. These usually do not last long, less than 20 minutes, but can last for a few hours. More rarely, migraine sufferers sometimes imagine that they can smell something. Others have reported that their whole body, or parts of their body, feel either very

Who Can be Helped by This Book

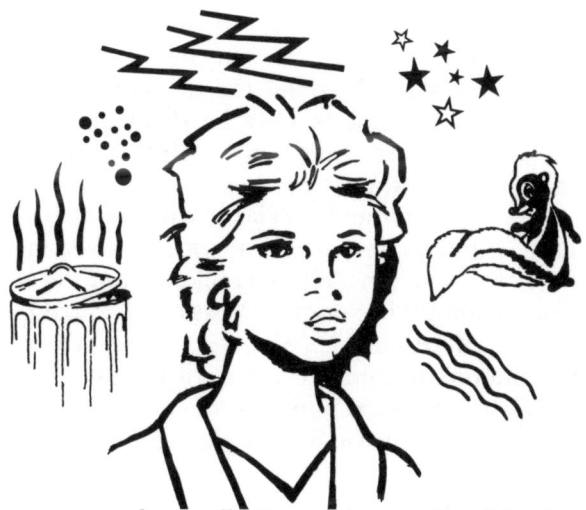

large or extremely small. One person who felt that her head was huge, light, and floating at the end of a long neck, said: 'I get all tired out from pulling my head down from the ceiling ... I've been pulling it down all night long'.

Lewis Carroll, in his famous book *Alice in Wonderland*, describes similar types of experiences: he suffered from migraine and it is often assumed that his descriptions are based upon his own migraine symptoms. Perhaps he, like many migraine sufferers, was afraid of being thought 'mad' if he wrote these things down in any form other than a fantastic story.

Lastly, you may experience feelings of having been in that exact same situation sometime before: *déjà vu* (already seen). Or quite the opposite, that everything seems strange or completely new to you: *jamais vu* (never seen).

> 'There would be my husband and children, just as usual, and in a flash they didn't seem to be quite the same. They were my husband and children all right – but they certainly weren't the same. There was something queer about it all. I felt as if I were standing on an inclined plane, looking down on them from a height of a few feet, watching myself serve breakfast ... I was not afraid, just amazed. I always knew I was really with them.'

Sometimes you may get feelings of general anxiety or fear, but these are less common, and may be your reaction to the symptoms rather than part of the headache itself.

All of these sensations may be difficult to admit to because you may feel that you will be labelled 'mad' or 'mentally ill'. The important thing is that these are fairly common accompaniments of classical migraine headaches. However, if they sometimes occur without a headache, you may be suffering from a type of epilepsy and the advice of your doctor should be sought. Occasionally during middle age the actual headaches become less severe or fail to develop, but the strange sensations still happen. In this case it will still be migraine. Indeed, changes in the type of sensation are not unusual over the lifetime of migraine sufferers.

Other symptoms typical of migraine

If you experience any of the strange type of sensations discussed above, then you do *not* suffer from tension headache, and it is probable that you have *classical* migraine attacks. Common migraine is similar to classical migraine, but without the aura. A 'text book' case of either type of migraine would have three further features. These are:

- Feeling sick or actually vomiting during the headache: some people have diarrhoea. This is why migraine is sometimes called sick headache.

- Throbbing pain that starts on one side of the head only. It may spread to the other side later. Pain on both sides of the head sometimes occurs in common migraine, however.

- A family history of similar headaches. Not all experts agree on this one.

Summary

To recap, migraine sufferers typically have some kind of warning that an attack is coming; there is often something specific that triggers the headache; they feel sick or vomit during it; the head pain is throbbing or pulsating and is generally only on one side of the head; and there may be a family history of similar headaches. Classical migraine sufferers also experience one or more 'strange sensations' before or during an attack.

In contrast, tension headaches have *none* of these features. Unlike migraine, the pain is like a tight pressure band around the head. Because tension headaches are so common (see Chapter 2), the odds are that if you suffer from them, someone in your family will also suffer from tension headaches. You can't call this a family history! Because migraines are less common and more distinct in their symptoms, it is more noticeable when they do run in families.

The Special Case of Cluster Headaches

Although cluster headache is supposed to be a type of migraine, its symptoms are so marked that it stands apart from classical and common types of migraine. Cluster headaches have none of the typical features of a migraine headache: no strange experiences, vomiting or specific triggers (although alcohol can occasionally set off attacks). Also, although migraine is much more common in women (see Chapter 2), cluster headache nearly always occurs in men between the ages of about 30 and 50. Some experts have noticed, oddly, that these men are often tall and smoke heavily!

Cluster headaches are so called because they occur in clusters. That is, when one occurs it is certain that many more will occur. People can be without a headache for a year and then have one every night for 6 to 12 weeks. Often the headaches are highly predictable; they can happen at the same time every night and some people have them at the same time each year. The pain is always very severe and feels like a stabbing in the back of the eye, generally only on one side of the head. Nothing can reliably relieve the pain. This is one kind of headache that really does drive men to tears. Actually, a streaming eye and a runny nose (on the side of the pain) are symptoms of this type of headache. Nevertheless, the pain is so severe that the occasional suicide has been reported. Unlike classical or common migraine, where the pain often forces people to lie quietly in darkness, cluster headache sufferers often cannot keep still. Some people have even banged their heads with the frustration and the pain.

Unfortunately, being a relatively uncommon condition, there have been no published accounts of the effects of self-treatments on cluster headache. For various reasons, you should perhaps be less optimistic if you suffer this kind of headache. On the bright side, however, it seems that often cluster headaches stop when the sufferer reaches middle-age.

Who Should Seek Further Help?

If you haven't already done so, it's best to seek your doctor's advice about your headaches, even if it's just to set your mind at rest. This is especially true if you are worried about what may be causing them. Worrying can make your headaches worse or more frequent. However, if your headaches have any of the following characteristics then you should *definitely* seek further medical advice:

Most Importantly...

- If your headaches are a new problem: that is, if they have started within the last few months.
- Especially if they began after a bang on the head, after starting medical treatment, or after you were involved in heavy exercise or a heated argument.

Or...

- If there have been any obvious changes in the intensity or in the symptoms associated with your headaches,
  particularly if you have recently begun to vomit.

Also...

- If your head pain is constant and never lets up.

- If your headaches have always been one-sided and always on the same side.

- If you have a fever with your headaches.

- If you are worried about your headaches.

If you *do* have any strange sensations or experiences at the same time as your headaches, other than the visual effects described in this chapter, then it is just as well to see your doctor. If you experience weakness, twitching, or numbness in your hands or feet, and especially if you have difficulty in speaking, then further investigation is wise. This is especially true if this is a recent development. Some people experience these effects as part of their migraine, but it is just as well to get it checked out.

If your headaches follow any of the above patterns, this does not necessarily mean that there is anything seriously wrong. Indeed, there may be a simple medical procedure that will alleviate your headaches. 'Better safe than sorry' is always a good motto to follow in health matters.

2. Learning about Headaches

What is Tension Headache?

The generally accepted explanation of tension headache is that it is caused by contraction of the muscles in the head and neck. That is why it is called *tension* headache, and why it is also called *muscle contraction* headache. When you tense your muscles in your arm for too long they soon start to ache; the same with the muscles in your head and neck. There are many reasons why the muscles become too tense. There obvious ones, like squinting or frowning for too long. Emotional tension can play a big part in adding to muscle tension. Poor posture or imbalances in the bone structure of the jaw, neck, shoulders or back can add extra tension to the muscles in the head and neck. Certain foods and drugs can also stop the body from relaxing (see Chapter 5). All of these things can combine to cause tension and fatigue in the relevant muscles, causing a headache.

Unfortunately this does not explain why some people get tension headaches regularly and some do not. It is definitely *not* because people who suffer these headaches are more emotionally uptight than those who do not. Nor do they generally have more bone structure imbalances, nor do they consume more stimulants, and so on. Some experts believe that we all react to stresses in our own way; Ms Jones may get stomach problems, Mr Smith may get asthma, and Ms Brown tension headaches. The idea is that Ms Jones' digestive system and Mr Smith's breathing system are both particularly prone to stress, and Ms Brown's muscular system in her head and neck is likewise. However, measurements of muscle tension seem to show that, in general, people who get tension headaches do not

Learning about Headaches

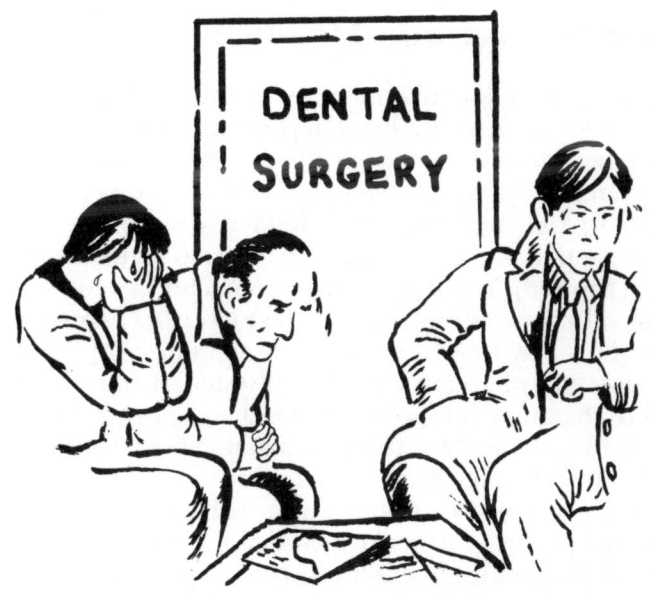

have especially reactive or tense head muscles. This means that something other than simple muscle tension must be causing the pain.

Some research has suggested that changes in the blood vessels in the head may cause the pain in tension headache. The blood vessels either shrink or swell – different studies have different findings. As you will see in the next section, this is probably the basis of migraine, so it fits in with the theory that migraine and tension headache are similar but differ only in how drastic the symptoms are. However, an alternative explanation of tension headache pain is that sufferers are just more sensitive to the effects of muscle tension. Not sensitive in an emotional sense, but in a physical sense. They don't have greater tension in general, but what they do have, they *feel* more, at least at the time of a headache. This idea of an increased sensitivity is explored in more depth in the section called 'Headache and Pain Control'.

What is Migraine Headache?

Many experts believe that migraine is caused by changes in the blood vessels in the head and neck. That is why it is sometimes called a *vascular* headache; 'vascular' means to do with the blood vessels. Migraine seems to happen in two stages. In the first stage the blood vessels to the head constrict – that is, they become narrower, so that less blood can get through. You'll remember from school biology that the blood provides oxygen and food to every part of the body. This may be why in classical migraine people have warning signs or an aura; the blood system does not serve parts of the brain very well, making them short of oxygen so 'switching them off' – or at least making them do their job poorly. In the case of the visual effects that often come before a migraine headache, it is probably the part of the brain that processes or makes sense of what you see that is affected. This is the generally accepted explanation for the strange experiences that go with migraine.

Recent research from Denmark has, however, suggested an alternative theory for the aura. This work has shown that a kind of damping down of the brain's activity spreads like a wave over the brain before a migraine. The brain is basically a bundle of millions of nerves that are connected; it seems that some nerves 'shut down' their operations and that this shutting down spreads to nerves nearby, and so on. This process has been called a *nerve storm*, but really it is just the opposite. These are new ideas, however, which need to be investigated further.

In the second stage of migraine, according to the traditional explanation, a lot of blood is forced through to areas of the head that had previously been deprived. Almost as if the body suddenly wakes up and realises that not enough blood is getting through to the parts that need it. Unfortunately, the blood system seems to overreact, forcing too much blood through. The arteries to the head become swollen and start to press on pain-sensitive areas, or become so stretched or dilated that they become painful themselves. Each heart-beat forces through more blood and as the extra blood comes through, the swollen vessels pulsate. That is why the pain in migraine is throbbing, and the pain seems to throb with your heart-beat.

There is a great deal of debate and controversy about what exactly happens in a migraine attack, and why some people get them while others don't. In some studies, blood flow measurements during a migraine have not shown the expected results; others have supported the two-stage theory. An important finding was that when migraine sufferers were given a chemical which narrows the blood vessels in the head, it did *not* cause an aura or a migraine attack. So it seems doubtful that a migraine is simply the blood system overreacting to the initial constriction of the vessels. Perhaps, as in tension headache, sufferers are more sensitive to changes in the blood vessels, or become more sensitive during the attack. This idea is discussed later in this chapter.

It is known, however, that the head muscles in migraine sufferers are often *more tense* than in tension headache sufferers. This may mean that muscle tension contributes to migraine. Perhaps the muscles, when they contract, narrow the blood vessels flowing through them so causing the first stage of migraine. Or it may just mean that migraine sufferers are particularly tense; not surprising really, given that the headaches are so painful and distressing. The idea of an emotionally tense 'migraine personality' is discussed later in this chapter.

Why do some people get migraine while others don't?

Most experts believe that some kind of chemical imbalance must be involved and that this imbalance probably occurs in the part of the nervous system called the *brainstem*. You will be meeting the brainstem again in the section on the body's system of pain control; it is the part of the brain that can stop you feeling pain. So anything going wrong there may make you feel pain more easily. Two chemicals in particular seem important in migraine attacks: *serotonin* and the *prostaglandins*. Serotonin has different functions in the body including helping to control pain and the control of blood vessel constriction. It is released into the bloodstream when particles in the blood called *platelets* stick together. Studies have shown more platelets sticking together and increased amounts of serotonin in a person's bloodstream before they have a migraine attack.

Prostaglandins also have many functions in the body. They may be important in migraine because, like serotonin, they control blood vessels. In addition, they influence how much blood platelets stick together and so how much serotonin is actually released. To complicate the picture, serotonin can in turn affect the amount of prostaglandins produced by the body. Scientific studies have shown raised levels of free fatty acids in the blood of migraine sufferers. The body uses these to make prostaglandins. When one kind of prostaglandin is given to people who do not normally suffer headaches then migraine-type headaches are often caused, sometimes complete with an aura. Ergotamine, a drug used to treat migraine, slows down the production of prostaglandins. It also does the same with serotonin, both directly and indirectly through lowering levels of prostaglandins. It seems likely, therefore, that imbalances of both the prostaglandins and serotonin are involved in migraine.

How do migraine sufferers develop whatever chemical imbalance causes on attack? It is likely that they are born with a vulnerability to this imbalance. As you will see later in this chapter, migraine can be passed down through families. This is not the whole story, however. If you are a migraine sufferer and are married to one then not all of your children will have the same problem. Whether or not they do depends on a number of things, not all of which are known. Among them are probably stress, hormone changes (both of which are dealt with later in this chapter), and sensitivities or allergies to foods and gases (see Chapter 7). It also seems that stress can cause or worsen these food sensitivities. All of these factors may affect the chemical imbalance in the brainstem, leading to the development of migraine. For instance, oestrogen (a female sex hormone that changes in amount during the menstrual cycle and is affected by contraceptive pills) influences both platelet activity, and therefore serotonin, and prostaglandin levels. However, some unfortunate people may be born with a chemical imbalance; migraine-like attacks have been observed in babies only a few months old. It is possible that these early attacks are set off by food sensitivities. Indeed, children who have tummy pains and vomiting can often go on to develop migraine when they are older.

Once a migraine is set off, the disorder seems to have a momentum of its own. For instance, in migraines that are triggered by the contraceptive pill, it often takes months for the headaches to stop once the person comes off the pill. Sometimes the headaches carry on plaguing the sufferer. Perhaps a vicious circle is set in motion. There is a theory that the worse the headaches get, the less the person can cope, both with the headaches and with life in general. Stress levels are increased, leading to worse headaches, and so on. However, with migraine, the vicious circle may also be chemical. Serotonin and the prostaglandins influence the production of each other, for instance. Another possibility is that an allergy of some kind may have been uncovered – this will be considered in more depth in Chapter 7.

Headache and Pain Control

Pain, like all sensations, is carried by nerves in the body. If you cut yourself, particular nerve endings or *receptors* in your skin start sending messages along the nerves to the spine and then up the spine to the brain. That is when you experience pain; your brain decides that it hurts. However, our bodies have developed an ingenious system for stopping the messages from getting through to our brain when it would be bad for us to feel pain. Pain is there for a purpose: to let us know that we are damaged so that we can do something about it. However, there are times when to feel pain might risk further damage; for instance, when we are facing or running away from danger. We would not put up a great fight or run very well if we were in agony. So the body needs a way of repressing pain at important times. It seems to have a very effective system for this. If you hurt yourself in a stressful situation like a traffic accident or even an important game of football, often you do not feel the pain until it is all over. Men wounded on the battlefield sometimes do not seem to feel pain. How does the body do this?

Messages are transmitted along nerves by a chemical process, and certain chemicals produced by the body called *neurotransmitters* determine whether the message gets through or not. Particular neurotransmitters are able to stop pain messages. They seem to do this mostly in the spinal cord. Experts now talk of a pain *gate* in the spinal cord. When it is 'open' pain messages are free to go up the spinal cord to the brain. When it is 'closed', you do not feel pain because the messages do not get through. This is because of these special neurotransmitters which are released: among these is our old friend serotonin. Perhaps the changes in the levels of serotonin that occur in migraine somehow leave the gate wide open, making the person feel pain when they normally would not. This may be the cause of the increased sensitivity to blood vessel changes and muscle tension that have been suggested as the basis for both tension and migraine headaches.

Recent research seems to show that the 'control centre' for the pain gate is in the part of the brain called the *brainstem*. This is the part of the nervous system at the top of the spine, underneath the main mass of the brain. In the brainstem chemicals can be produced that are very similar to morphine, which is an effective drug for pain control. These chemicals are called *endorphins*. It appears that the brainstem opens and closes the pain gate in the spinal cord by means of these endorphins. Morphine also has its effect by closing the gate. Some scientists believe that low levels of endorphins, leaving the gate open, lead to the increased sensitivity that lies behind both migraine and tension headaches. It is possible that both the endorphins and serotonin are involved in this process.

What is most interesting for the person looking for self-help methods for reducing their headaches, however, are methods for getting the brainstem to close the gate. Anxiety seems to open the gate; relaxation closes it. In the following section the links between stress, relaxation and headaches will be explored further. More importantly, low stress levels together with dietary changes may ensure that the chemical imbalance is corrected so that the gate is not opened unnecessarily in the first place.

Stress, Headaches and Relaxation

What is stress?

Stress is not something that happens to you, like losing a job or the ending of a relationship. Rather, it is your reaction to an event or situation. An event is only stressful if it produces a certain reaction in you. That reaction is partly psychological or emotion (you feel harassed, upset, angry, and so on) and partly physical. Sometimes the reaction can be wholly physical; your body is stressed yet you do not feel uptight or under pressure. The details of the physical part of the stress reaction are too complex to go into here. The main changes are similar to the kind of changes your body undergoes when you are anxious. If you are in this state for a long while then your body becomes stressed.

There are times when we need to be keyed up for action; this is the purpose of anxiety. You may have noticed certain symptoms when you are very anxious: your heart beating faster, sweaty palms, dry mouth, rapid shallow breathing, and so on. All of these symptoms are under the automatic control of part of our nervous system called the *autonomic* nervous system. They are signs of what is called *autonomic arousal* – meaning that your autonomic nervous system is 'turning itself up'. It does this when you are very excited or angry, not only when you are anxious. Chemical messengers or *hormones*, the most important of which is *adrenalin*, are carried in the blood to tell the body what to do. These messengers tell your body to divert blood away from the organs that do not need it and into the muscles and brain, so that you become ready for action. Your muscles are also told to tense up for the same purpose.

It is these changes in the blood and muscle systems that are often thought important for understanding how stress is linked to headaches. However, the stress reaction is caused by changes in the blood chemistry, and recent thinking is that these changes might be the real culprits in headaches.

When you are uptight your autonomic system 'turns itself up', producing adrenalin and other messengers to prepare you for action. The trouble is, often we get uptight when we don't need to do something physical, so these substances stay around in our systems without being 'burned off' and may cause mischief. That is probably why physical exercise can help to reduce stress build-up. This is discussed more in Chapter 6.

Stress and headaches

So part of the stress reaction is a change in the blood system and increased levels of muscle tension. You may now have an idea why both migraine and tension headaches are linked to stress. It is perhaps clearest in the case of tension headache. More stress means greater muscle contraction, and if a person is particularly sensitive to tension in the head or neck, then pain is likely. In fact, things are probably much more complicated than this. The reason why a person becomes more sensitive to muscular tension is not simple, and may have to do with the opening of the pain gate. The pain gate may itself be opened by substances as part of the stress reaction. It is also likely that people get stuck in vicious circles. The worse the pain, the more they tense up against it, the more pain they get, and so on. The worse the headache, the less they can cope with everyday stress, the greater the tension, the worse the headache. The same circles may also happen in migraine.

As far as the connection between stress and migraine is concerned, experts are much more at odds with each other. Stress might cause the first stage of migraine, in which the blood vessels to the head and neck constrict. This may be part of the stress reaction itself. Unfortunately some studies show that these blood vessels narrow when the person is stressed while other studies show that they widen. Other studies show no reaction! The problem is that it is difficult to produce stress in a scientific study because different people are stressed by different things. Anything that is stressful to everyone would have to be something pretty awful and it would be wrong to put innocent people through it for the sake of an experimental study.

What may be more relevant than the reaction of blood vessels to stress is the changes in blood chemistry. As we have seen, simply causing the blood vessels to constrict in people who suffer from migraine does not necessarily set off a headache. So blood vessel changes in the first stage of migraine are only part of the story. It is likely that stress causes an imbalance in blood chemistry, which then leads to both changes in the blood vessels and the increased sensitivity that causes head pain. This chemical imbalance may also lead to other symptoms of migraine, such as the aura and feeling sick.

The long-term effects of continual stress may also cause headaches over and above 'one-off' events that are stressful. In the case of tension headache, it may be that sufferers have particular difficulty in getting rid of muscular tension so that a build-up is more likely. The same may be true of migraine sufferers. Also, in long-term stress there tends to be a build-up in the blood of hormones and other substances, particularly those related to adrenalin. With high levels of muscle tension *and* stress hormones, it is no surprise that comparatively insignificant events can then seem to trigger a headache; the proverbial 'straw that broke the camel's back'.

Are all headaches stress-related?

This is a difficult if not impossible question to answer. It seems unlikely that all tension headaches have the same causes and mechanisms, and that all migraine headaches have likewise. Often there can be many different causes of a problem, but one end result or *final common pathway*. It may be that allergies, chemicals in foods, the stress reaction and so on can *all* set the final common pathway in motion, either on their own or in combination with each other. In the case of migraine, the final common pathway may be an imbalance of serotonin in the brainstem or the swelling of blood vessels in the head. In tension headache, it may be an increased sensitivity to the sustained contraction of the muscles in the head and neck. It is the final common pathway that leads to a headache but it is important to see that many things can set it in motion. The various influences may have to add together, or some may be enough on their own.

When one thing on its own is sufficient to set the final common pathway in motion, the sufferer may notice a link. If a person realises that nervous tension triggers a headache, then stress is such a factor *for that person*. However, this does not mean that for people who discover *no* link, stress is not one of the underlying causes of their headaches. Perhaps stress is insufficient on its own, but when added to something else, may cause a headache – and if the stress were removed then the headache would not occur. Many people also 'bury' their tension so that on the surface they are calm and relaxed but underneath they are uptight. They may not even admit it to themselves. This may be particularly true for those who see themselves as 'cool' and in control: businessmen take note! If the person were like this, even though stress may be an underlying cause of their headaches, they would not recognise the link because they would not recognise the stress.

Often people who have not noticed a link between stress and their headaches discover one by completing a *headache diary* over a period of time. This is because especially stressful events may not in themselves cause a headache, but a build-up of tension or continual stress may be more relevant. That is why it is best to record both emotional tension and all upsetting or unusual events in the diary. Chapter 4 gives more details on this. For instance, one recent study showed that there was a direct link between stressful life events such as moving house, getting married, and so on, and the frequency and severity of migraine.

You may now understand how stress may be an underlying cause of your headaches, even when there is no obvious link. Either the build-up is important, or stress is an insufficient cause on its own but adds to other things to set off a headache. The last thing to remember when you wonder whether all headaches are stress-related is that *learning to relax* generally reduces headaches. This has been proven in many studies with both migraine and tension headache cases, and often the improvements are better than those achieved by drugs. This again implies that stress plays a part in both migraine and tension headaches.

Relaxation and headaches

You may now have some ideas about how learning relaxation techniques can help reduce headaches. If a person is more relaxed, their background levels of stress will be lower: when another trigger comes along and adds to the background level of stress the chances of setting off a headache will be less. Also, deliberately relaxing will stop a build-up of tension or stress. Lastly, it is possible to use relaxation techniques to stop the first stage of a headache when the person feels one coming on. In migraine, the person may avoid the initial constriction of the blood vessels in the head and the built-up of certain substances in the bloodstream by relaxing. In tension headache the tension-pain vicious circle could be broken. Even if these attempts were not wholly successful, the degree to which the blood vessels narrow, and the degree to which the muscles tense up against the pain can both be reduced. Relaxation techniques can therefore both reduce the number of headaches and lower their intensity.

The 'Headache Personality'

There have been many myths and misunderstandings about what kind of people suffer headaches. This is particularly true with migraine sufferers. People who get migraine headaches are supposed to be tense, driving personalities who are set in their ways, find it difficult to change, and who cannot express their feelings. They have to do everything 'just so', are always on time and always organised. They get upset if their house is the least bit untidy, or if their work does not meet their own very high standards. 'Rigid' and 'perfectionist' are two words that are often used to describe the so-called migraine personality.

It is true that some people who suffer from migraine are like this. However, many are not and scientific studies have shown that this kind of personality is not vastly more common among migraine sufferers than among people in general. The evidence for a 'tension headache personality' is non-existent; it is unlikely even that they are more tense than other people.

The idea of a migraine personality has come from psychoanalytic theories about headaches. Psychoanalysis is a school of psychology started by Sigmund Freud which suggests that many physical and psychological symptoms are due to underlying emotional conflicts that the person is not aware of. Various psychoanalysts have, for instance, suggested that headaches are a symptom of unexpressed anger. A person may have a lot of anger about something but is afraid to express it. Perhaps someone is afraid to express anger toward a partner in case he or she leaves. In this case it is a conflict between anger and fear of being abandoned. To avoid the conflict, people may unwittingly force it into unconsciousness, so that they are no longer aware of the conflict or the anger. And it comes out as headaches. Other psychoanalysts have suggested various other conflicts may be the cause of headaches, including ones to do with sex and forbidden desires. Once you think that one particular conflict is the root of all headaches, then the jump to the idea that all headache sufferers have a similar personality is not so absurd.

It may be true that some people's headaches are caused by unconscious conflicts. However, very often the conflict will not be unconscious. A woman who has to bite her tongue for fear of releasing her husband's anger may well be aware that she has to leave her anger unexpressed. This probably has its effect on her headaches only because it is yet another source of stress, rather than being any special cause in itself.

Who gets Headaches?

In a group of ten women, on average three or four would suffer frequent or severe headaches; out of a group of ten men, probably two or three. Only about one in ten in both of these groups would be totally immune. Headaches can occur in any social class and in any job or at any income level. Tension headaches seem to be as frequent in men as in women, but migraine is probably about three times more common in women. Part of the reason for this is the fact that migraine headaches are often linked to menstrual periods and the contraceptive pill; this subject will be dealt with in the next section. It is not known whether more women than men suffer migraine when those who suffer menstrual- and pill-related headaches are excluded. It is probable that women *are* more vulnerable, because it seems as though oestrogens, one of the female hormones, are involved in migraine.

If someone in your family has headaches, what are the chances that you will suffer them too? This is a difficult question to answer. Tension headache is so common that the chances are that you will suffer from them anyway, at least occasionally. With migraine, it seems that at least 50%

of migraine sufferers have close relatives who also suffer similar headaches. This is opposed to 5 – 10% of the relatives of a headache-free person. However, headaches are not simply inherited. Identical twins, who have the same genetic make-up, do not always both develop migraine. It seems that other influences affect whether or not someone actually develops migraine, even if they are born vulnerable to it. Some of these influences are probably to do with the amount of stress in a person's life and how it is dealt with. Food sensitivities may also play a part. Another important factor is variation in hormone levels.

Women, hormones and migraine

Migraine-type headaches are much more common in women than men, but this is not true as far as children are concerned. Some experts believe that hormone changes are responsible for this difference, and that oestrogens, the female sex hormones, are probably somehow involved in causing migraines. There are many other facts that support this idea.

First, migraines are often linked to the menstrual cycle, during which there are large hormone changes. It was originally thought that the increase in the blood levels of progesterone (the other female sex hormone) was a cause of this, but recent evidence points to the sharp drop in oestrogen levels. One study found that seven out of ten women said that at least some of their headaches were linked to their periods. Many of these headaches may be due to the extra emotional tension some women feel just before their periods on top of the hormone changes. It is possible that hormone changes are important to *all* women with migraine and are merely more noticeable in those whose headaches are linked to their periods.

Secondly, contraceptive pills, which contain oestrogen, often trigger migraine attacks. It is unfortunately not yet known whether low-oestrogen pills are better in this regard. Thirdly, female sufferers rarely have a migraine when they are pregnant, when there are increases in oestrogen and especially progesterone, but the levels of these hormones in the blood stay fairly steady. Lastly, migraines generally tail off when a woman reaches her menopause, the point at which the regular change in her hormones finish; and oestrogen replacement therapy sometimes causes headaches!

Exactly how hormone changes cause migraines is not certain, but it may have something to do with the effects on the brainstem; as we have seen, oestrogen can upset the balance of both serotonin and the prostaglandins. However, some specialists believe that headaches due to these causes are a separate kind of headache from other migraines, so that hormones may not be relevant to all migraines. Indeed, some women think that their menstrual headaches feel different from their other migraines. There is not a great deal of evidence to support this theory, however.

3. The Medical Approach

Are Headaches a Medical Problem?

It should be obvious from the previous chapter that there are many things that can cause headaches. Few of the causes of headache are physical, in the sense that there is something wrong with your body. Very occasionally there is a physical cause for someone's headaches, high blood pressure perhaps, or something more serious such as a brain tumour. That is why somebody suffering from headaches should always see their doctor and have a thorough medical examination to rule out physical causes. This is not to say that *how* you get a headache is not physical. On the contrary, disturbances in the blood chemistry, excessive muscle tension, and swollen blood vessels are all physical. However, the causes of these disturbances are generally *environmental*: what you eat, how you react to stressful situations, taking the pill, and so on. They are environmental in the sense that they are to do with the 'outside world' and the way that you think and act, rather than anything wrong with your body. So most of the causes of headache are not physical. Even most hormone changes are natural changes, not an illness or disease. So if we are going to treat headaches sensibly – by dealing with the causes – then medical treatment is not generally the best way.

It may also be obvious from the last chapter that scientists do not yet know the complete picture of *how* a headache happens – its mechanisms. There is a lot of research evidence that enables us to make educated guesses about the main mechanisms. However, nothing is certain and the fine details are certainly not known. When the mechanisms of headaches are fully understood – particularly the final common pathways that were discussed in the previous

The Medical Approach

chapter – then perhaps a medical 'cure' will be obvious. But at present medical treatment involves the suppression of the symptoms of headache, rather than providing a cure. It makes more sense to deal with the causes – it is healthier in the long run too. If you don't treat the causes of persistent headaches then you may find that other kinds of problems emerge. For instance, if you are under a lot of stress and your headaches are suppressed by taking drugs, it would not be surprising if other more serious illnesses emerged. That is why the treatments in this book are aimed at the various *causes* of headaches.

Many people do not share this viewpoint. They see headaches as a medical problem and go to their doctor expecting to be treated with drugs. As you will read in the rest of this chapter, drugs can be of some help. But they are perhaps best seen as a way of 'turning the tide' against headaches, of 'getting you back on your feet', rather than a permanent solution. There are better, more effective ways of beating many kinds of headaches in the long run – by dealing with the causes. Your doctor may offer you drugs but may also be pleased to hear that you are trying to tackle the cause of your headaches for yourself. If the doctor seems rather sceptical about your intentions – don't be put off. All of the treatment suggestions in this book are supported by research evidence.

The most important reason for going to your doctor is to rule out any medical causes. Then, if they are sympathetic, to receive advice and guidance on the medical implications of anything that you try – a special diet, for instance, or relaxation exercises. If they are not sympathetic then don't worry because all of the things suggested in this book are harmless if followed correctly. Professional guidance is always worthwhile, however, particularly where diets are concerned. Addresses where you can find specialist guidance are given at the end of this book.

If your doctor fails to find a physical cause or proper drug treatment for your headaches, he or she may conclude that they are 'psychological'. You may even be referred for psychotherapy. This does not necessarily mean that it is all in your mind. Often, depression or anxiety can exacerbate your headaches or even start them (see Chapter 6). Emotional problems are a tremendous source of stress, and psychotherapy can help you deal with this. However, it is *not* your doctor's responsibility to make you better. It is *yours*. It is *your* problem, *your* pain, and *your* thoughts and behaviour that may be causing your headaches.

Taking an active role in treatment

Once you have accepted that it is your responsibility to help yourself get better, taking a more active role follows naturally. So ask questions. Learn about your problem. Read this whole book from cover to cover. A short list of recommended reading is also included at the end of this book. Don't sit back and wait for your doctor to prescribe treatment. Suggest things yourself, perhaps from this book. Ask for guidance if you think that there may possibly be medical complications. Try as many different approaches as you can. Keep trying until you find something that works. Don't get dispirited if the first approach does not pay dividends – the next one may. The more things you try out (as long as you do them properly) the more chance you have of beating the problem.

Since you may have been offered drug treatment by your doctor and you probably have taken tablets for your headaches in the past, you will want to know about the various kinds of drugs that are available. If you are ready to assume responsibility for your problem, you will need to know the pros and cons of taking drugs, their benefits and their drawbacks. That is the only way of deciding if they are right for you. Remember, however, that prescribing the correct doses, being aware of any interactions with other medications, and so on, is your doctor's job – and not an easy one.

Painkillers (Analgesics)

Painkillers suppress symptoms but do not deal with the actual cause of the headache. For people who suffer only occasional headaches this is the most convenient option. They can also be useful in making life more bearable when a person is trying to do without more powerful medications. Unfortunately there is some evidence that long-term use of painkillers can actually impair the body's own system of pain control (see Chapter 2), as well as sometimes leading to dangerous side-effects. So you would do well to use them only occasionally.

There is an extra complication with taking painkillers for migraine headaches. When you feel nauseous (and especially if you are sick), your stomach is not working properly, so that any medicine that you take will not be completely absorbed. So it is always best to take *soluble* painkillers, which are much more easily absorbed. This also reduces the risk of unpleasant side-effects on your digestive system. Migraine sufferers may like to try taking a *combination* drug: a painkiller combined with a drug that helps your stomach to work better and so reduce the nausea. Migravess and Paramax are two examples, but they are only available on prescription from a doctor. You may find that because your body now absorbs the painkiller more effectively, the combination drug may be much more effective than just a painkiller on its own. This way, you may be able to avoid taking the more dangerous drugs sometimes prescribed for migraine, such as ergotamine. The main painkillers are all available from a chemist without a prescription. They are:

Aspirin This has not turned out to be the safe drug that was once thought. Although an effective painkiller, aspirin can cause irritation, ulcers, and bleeding in a person's digestive system if taken frequently. Taking it after meals can help reduce this. Other possible side-effects include ringing in the ears (tinnitus), skin reactions, and bronchial problems.

Paracetamol This can also be an effective painkiller but again you should beware of taking it regularly. Similar irritation (although much less than with aspirin) of the digestive system can result, and possible liver damage with excessive use.

Ibuprofen This has recently become available without prescription on both sides of the Atlantic, and was originally developed in the treatment of arthritis. It is a powerful painkiller but like all drugs is not without side-effects, although these seem to be fairly uncommon. Do not take ibuprofen if you have suffered from peptic ulcers, kidney or heart problems, or an allergy to aspirin in the past. Also, do not take it if you are taking any other type of medication unless your doctor gives you express permission.

Caffeine This is a stimulant that is an ingredient in many painkillers that can be bought at a chemist, e.g. Solpadeine. It can make you feel better in the short term for two reasons: by giving you artificial energy and by narrowing the blood vessels to the head, thereby reducing pain if these are involved in your headache. However, caffeine can also worsen your headaches in the long run. Being a stimulant, it increases both nervous tension and muscle tension, making the next headache more likely. This is true for both migraine and tension headaches. Some specialists also believe that *rebound* headaches are likely after taking caffeine. This can happen if, as a result of taking drugs, the blood vessels in your head have narrowed, and then when the drug wears off the blood vessels expand, sometimes past their normal size. If you remember, this is one of the causes of the pain in migraine. Thus another headache is caused, and if you take the caffeine-containing medication for this one, you are caught in a vicious circle.

Drugs used specifically for migraine

These drugs are only available on prescription from a doctor. They may be divided into three categories. First, there are the drugs used for stopping an attack from developing into a full-blown headache. Second, there are drugs used to alleviate the nausea and sickness that often accompany migraine, and lastly there are the drugs that are used for preventing attacks.

Ergotamine This is the main drug given to abort migraine attacks, although caffeine is also often recommended. Ergotamine is a powerful drug that is available in several different forms and is contained in medicines such as Cafergot and Migril. If taken early enough, it can abort a migraine attack and can even be helpful in some cluster headaches. There are many problems with this drug, however, if it is taken frequently. There is evidence that in the long run it actually *causes* migraines. It also works partly by shrinking the blood vessels, so rebound headaches are likely. Some experts believe that people can develop a sensitivity to ergotamine in the same way that some people are sensitive to certain foods, which again can lead to extra migraines. It is difficult to say whether these 'sensitivity' headaches are simply rebound headaches. Either way, it is apparent that taking ergotamine frequently can contribute to a migraine problem, even though in the short term it provides relief. People can then get caught in a similar vicious circle to the one caused by caffeine. There can be strong withdrawal effects when the person tries doing without ergotamine. Among these withdrawal effects are severe rebound headaches, so people think that they cannot do without the drug.

One of the biggest problems is over-use of ergotamine. This can be due to the rebound headache vicious circle but can also occur with people who suffer frequent migraines anyway. There is an irresistible temptation when you are in agony to take tablets to achieve some kind of relief. Or to take tablets to abort an attack when you have something important to do that day. These temptations are strong no matter how many tablets you have taken in the recent past. Some people even take ergotamine on a regular basis to prevent migraines. *On no account* do this – it is dangerous. There is a limit, and a fairly low one, as to how much medication you can take. One manufacturer's data sheet says that no more than four tablets in one attack and no more than six in one week is the limit. Check with your doctor. The side-effects from over-use are serious and can include severe muscle pains, gangrene of the fingers and toes, mental confusion, fits, paralysis, and (ironically) severe headaches and nausea. Even moderate use may still leave you feeling sick and very tired for some time after the attack – some people put this down to the migraine attack itself. Other side-effects can be diarrhoea, drowsiness, cramps and numbness. All in all, ergotamine is best reserved for those people who suffer only occasional migraines. Definitely do not take it if you have had a history of heart problems or peptic ulcers. One-third of migraine sufferers who are treated with drugs take this one, which suggests that it may be over-prescribed.

Metaclopramide This is the most common medication taken to reduce vomiting and feelings of nausea. Tablets such as Maxolon and Primperan are forms of metaclopramide. It is also available in combination with painkillers such as aspirin and paracetamol, since it may improve the absorption of these. The side-effects from metaclopramide can include constipation, drowsiness, and sometimes more serious effects such as finding it difficult to walk properly.

Non-steroid anti-inflammatory drugs (otherwise known as NSAIDs!) These were developed for the treatment of rheumatism and arthritis, but recently one of them, naproxen, has been shown to be of some use in the treatment of migraine. It can be used for both the treatment of single attacks, and for preventing migraine. Side-effects include water retention and irritation of the digestive system.

The Medical Approach

Other preventative drugs

These are generally taken daily to prevent migraine attacks. This does not mean you will be taking them forever, because they can be used for interrupting vicious circles. As we have seen in the previous chapter, people often get caught in a vicious circle of headaches leading to more emotional tension leading to more headaches. And as we have discussed above, taking drugs that work by shrinking the blood vessels can create vicious circles of their own. So preventing migraines for a few months may be enough to break these vicious circles, enabling you then to tackle them with self-help methods. However, as with all drug treatment, you will have to balance the side-effects and possible dangers with the benefits.

Methysergide, otherwise known as *Desaril*. This is said to be the most effective preventative treatment for migraine, but it also produces some of the worst side-effects. It is related to ergotamine, and like that drug can lead to severe headaches when it is withdrawn. It can produce fibrous tissue inside the abdomen and the heart if taken over long periods. It can also lead to kidney and liver problems, nausea, dizziness and drowsiness. For these reasons it should only be used as a last resort. The side-effects can be minimised by taking it for three-month periods, separated by at least one month.

Beta-blockers This group of drugs was developed for the treatment of high blood pressure and some heart diseases, and has also been used for anxiety problems. They help prevent migraines in about 50% of cases. The most useful beta-blockers are propanolol, metoprolol and acebutolol. The most marked side-effects are cold hands and feet and exhaustion due to the lowered blood pressure – you should not take these if you already have poor circulation. Disturbed sleep is also a complaint. The beta-blockers may set off asthma attacks if you suffer from these, and the risk of heart failure may also be increased.

Pizotifen, prescribed as Sanomigran or BC-105. This preventative drug is about as effective as the beta-blockers. Side-effects include feeling tired and drowsy, and rapid weight gain. It seems to increase the appetite of some people, which can worsen the weight gain considerably; if it is taken at bedtime then this risk is lessened.

Clonidine, known also as Dixarit. This was once thought to be useful in preventing migraine attacks, but recent research has not confirmed its effectiveness. Nevertheless, it is still widely prescribed and some migraine sufferers find it very effective.

Drugs used specifically for tension headache

Tranquillisers Although painkillers are by far the most widely used drugs in the treatment of tension headache, doctors will often prescribe tranquillisers if the problem is severe. These can reduce both nervous tension and muscle tension, so helping tension headaches. The different kinds of tranquillisers are too numerous to mention, but perhaps the most common are the *benzodiazepines*. These include the frequently-prescribed *diazepam*, also called Valium. They can be of great value in the short term, but over a period of time complications can set in. There is a distinct danger of addiction, with often quite alarming withdrawal effects. So, again, they are perhaps best used for breaking the tension headache – more tension vicious circle.

People often complain of feeling 'druggy' or 'spaced out' on benzodiazepines. Exhaustion and severe depression can also occur. Lastly, it can be very dangerous to combine these tranquilisers with alcohol or with sleeping tablets. Learning relaxation techniques is probably more effective, and without side-effects.

Antidepressants These are occasionally prescribed for tension headaches. Sometimes it is thought that depression underlies headaches (see Chapter 6), so that helping the depression will ease the headaches. There may also be a more direct action on the headaches themselves. Antidepressants may also be taken for migraine for similar reasons.

The most common group of drugs prescribed are the *tricyclics*, among which amitriptyline has been used for both migraine and tension headaches. They may also help with reducing muscle tension and may also have a more specific effect on the chemicals in the brain. However, antidepressants have their own dangers and side-effects, which can include a constant dry mouth and constipation. Again, it is dangerous to combine these drugs with alcohol or with sedatives.

Summary

Apart from painkillers, the drugs used for migraine are different from those used for tension headaches. Some are prescribed for both kinds of headaches, though, and in general it is not known *how* drugs work. There also seems to be an incredible variation in what is effective for any one individual. This suggests that there may be many different underlying causes for headaches, although the presenting symptoms may be the same. The symptoms would correspond to the final common pathway that was discussed in the previous chapter. Unfortunately, it is not known as yet how to match the correct medication to an individual, beyond the headache diagnosis. So expect a trial-and-error approach from your doctor, and don't get too dispirited or angry if you are on your fifth kind of medication. It is (probably) not your doctor's fault!

Reading through this list of the drugs used in the treatment of headache, you may be struck by the number and severity of the side-effects that are possible. Of course, with adequate supervision these will be minimised and serious side-effects should be rare. However, the risks *do* exist. If you are prescribed *any* drugs by your doctor, ask about the side-effects and risks. Be bold – it's *your* choice. It is up to you whether you feel that the pros will outweigh the cons, and you cannot decide this if you are not in possession of the facts.

Beware, in general, of any long-term drug treatment; if this is needed then you should definitely consider the kinds of self-help approaches put forward in this book. One study showed that as many as four out of ten headache sufferers experience marked improvements after all drugs were discontinued for two to three days. *Always* withdraw, however, using your doctor's advice – this is especially true with preventative drugs for migraine, many of which can lead to heart problems with sudden withdrawal. Perhaps medication is best used as a short-term fillip, so that any vicious circles can be broken, enabling you to then use a more 'wholesome' approach.

4. Recording Your Headaches

This chapter will explain how to make a detailed record of your headaches in the form of a *headache diary*. There is no set way of doing this and how you do it will depend on the exact information you need. You may want to know first why making such a record is important, and exactly what it can tell you.

A Record is Important

Keeping a record of your headaches is important because it can give you information that will help you to understand your problem. This information may also give clues as to ways in which you can reduce your headaches. Keeping a proper record will make clear what causes or makes your headaches worse. You may think you already know this – after all, you may have been suffering from them for many years. However, it is amazing how many people discover new facts after completing a headache diary over a period of time.

The second reason for keeping a proper record of your headaches is to keep tabs on the effects of any form of treatment. Some treatments, like learning relaxation techniques, take some while to work; and when they do work, they do so gradually. Because change is slow, major improvements over a period of months may be missed completely until reference is made to a diary. Some people think:

> 'Well ... if the improvement is not obvious then it's not worth carrying on with the treatment ... so there's no point in keeping a detailed record'.

The point is, people often do not notice 'obvious' improvements. A drop from, say, 18 to 8 headaches a month over a period of a few months may not be noticed or may be underestimated. This is because memory fades, and because people tend to focus on recent unpleasant experiences. However, such a change can have a major impact on somebody's life: ten extra headache-free days a month! It is important to be able to see in black and white the gains that have been made so that morale is kept up. This is especially true for treatments that you have to work at, and for treatments in which change is gradual, like the one described in the next chapter. Of course, if the headache diary shows no benefits, then that is equally important to know and another approach can be tried.

Keeping a Headache Diary

You will have to decide two things before you keep a headache diary:

- what information you need

- how you are going to collect it.

What information do you need?

You need to record both your headaches and whatever is likely to affect them. The most important thing to record apart from your headaches is *emotional tension* or how *uptight* you are. You may not consider this relevant to your headaches, but it is likely to play a part in most migraine and tension headaches. Chapter 2 went over this in some detail. Try charting levels of emotional tension and see if there is a link to your headaches. Emotional tension can mean many different things, and you will have to decide in advance what it means as far as your diary is concerned – guidelines for this are in the next section.

Other things you need to record are:

- *Your periods*, if you are a woman. Headaches are often linked to the menstrual cycle, although this may not be obvious to you. It is probably advisable for all women to include this in their diaries. Unfortunately, however, it will be many months before you can discern a pattern.
- *Possible triggers*. The most common ones for migraine headache were listed in Chapter 1, and the ones you should definitely include are given later in this chapter. The special subject of foods is discussed in Chapter 7. There are no specific triggers for tension headaches. As the name implies, they are usually linked to general emotional tension.
- *Events* of a stressful, upsetting, or unusual nature. Sometimes when something happens you may not feel particularly stressed or upset yet it may still set off a headache.
- *Associated symptoms*. This will be most useful when you are trying to decide what kind of headache you are suffering from. The most common symptoms that accompany both tension and migraine headaches were listed in Chapter 1 (see especially Table 1). You may like to use the symptom checklist given later in this chapter.
- *Medication*. Use this as another indicator of how well a treatment programme is working. Most medications have side-effects, some of which are unpleasant (see Chapter 3). If a treatment reduces the need for tablets, even if the headaches are not reduced, then perhaps it will be worth persevering with it.

How to collect the information

First you will need to decide whether you are going to keep a separate diary or whether you will be keeping your records in a diary that you already keep. Since you need to write in it four times each day, it is best to keep it with you throughout the day. Don't be tempted to look back over the day, and fill it in that evening or the next day. There have been many studies to show that people are not very good at remembering accurately their pain or emotional state. Because you will have to keep it with you all day, some people try and incorporate it in their present diary. This is fine if there is space; you will have to make sure that special columns for your records are drawn in, in advance. If you are a habitual diary checker then this will remind you to keep your headache record. Equally, having a separate diary or notepad for your headaches may act as a reminder if you keep it in a well-used pocket or in your handbag or purse.

What does a headache diary look like?

The simpler the better! You will need separate columns for everything that you are recording. This will be at least:

PAIN. Perhaps two columns
EMOTIONAL TENSION

and may include:

PERIOD DAYS
TRIGGERS
EVENTS
SYMPTOMS
MEDICATION

How you can record each of these is discussed next. You will have to record everything four times a day: at *breakfast, lunch, supper*, and *bedtime*. So this means *four rows* for each day. Your diary will look something like this:

Recording your Headaches

Day/Date	Pain	Tension	Period	Triggers	Events	Symptoms	Medication
Monday 8th July							
Tuesday 9th July							
Wednesday 10th July							
Thursday 11th July							
Friday 12th July							

What goes in each of these squares? That depends on what you are recording:

PAIN

Somehow, you will have to 'measure' your pain. The simplest way is to rate your pain on a scale of 0 (meaning no pain at all) to 10 (meaning the worst headache I have ever had). So, a bad headache may be 7 or 8, a moderate headache 4 or 5, and so on. With this method, you only have to leave space for one number.

Alternatively, you may like to measure two aspects of your pain. Firstly, how *intense* your headache is: this would go from 0 (meaning again no pain at all) to 10 (meaning the most intense headache I have ever had). So, a pretty intense headache may be 6 or 7, a mild headache may be 2 or 3, and so on. The second aspect you could measure is *how much the pain bothers you*. At first thought, this may seem the same thing. But just think of the times when you have just had to get on with life while having a blinder of a headache. Because you have other more important things on your mind, the pain doesn't seem to bother you as much.

However, once you stop, the pain can become overwhelming. To measure this aspect of your headache, you can rate it from 0 (meaning not bothersome in the least) to 10 (meaning totally overwhelming). This can be useful information because some treatments affect how you cope with your pain as well as the pain itself. This will be discussed in Chapter 6. If you do decide to record both aspects of your headache pain, then you will need space for two columns of numbers.

Remember, record your pain *only* at the specified times. Don't be tempted if your headache is wearing off to think back an hour or two when it was really bad and put down that reading. Record how your headache is at the time. Don't worry, over a period of a month or so, it will produce a more accurate picture than if you are continually thinking back or if you only record your headaches at their worst.

EMOTIONAL TENSION

You can measure emotional tension in a similar way, using numbers. However, emotional tension can mean lots of things; it can mean being angry, worried, excited, under pressure, or simply being in a tense situation. What we are after here is the kind of tension that makes you feel *uptight* or *under stress*. Say you have had an argument during the afternoon. If you are the type of person who 'explodes' and lets it all out in an argument, by dinner you may be completely relaxed, and score perhaps 0 or 1. If on the other hand you tend to 'bottle things up' and mull things over, by dinner you might be even more uptight than during the argument, and score 8 or 9. So even though the situation may appear relaxed, inside you are feeling stressed or uptight. You can measure this type of emotional tension on a scale of 0 to 10, with 0 meaning completely relaxed and 10 meaning the most tense or uptight that I have ever felt. Again, only record your tension at the specified times.

YOUR PERIODS

Note down the days on which you have your period. A separate column is not necessary here (you can make a note by the date) but having one will remind you to keep a record.

TRIGGERS

This column is particularly important for those people who suspect that some or all of their headaches are migraine. First, make a list of everything that you think may possibly cause headaches. *Always* include the following:

- Oversleeping or a poor night's sleep
- Physical exertion or exercise
- Bright lights or glare
- Loud noise
- Hunger
- Alcohol, especially red wine
- Cheese, oranges and chocolate
- Coffee

and perhaps other foods or any other trigger that you suspect may cause your headaches. Look at the list in Chapter 1 and the discussion on foods in Chapter 7 for ideas. You can have one thick column for all these triggers and then simply write in whenever you have experienced one in the meantime. It would be clearer if you decided on some kind of shorthand; for instance, A for alcohol, G for glare, CS for cheese, CT for chocolate, and so on. Then you would have room if two or more triggers coincided. Of course, if after a few weeks you decide that something is definitely not linked to your headaches, you can stop recording it and perhaps introduce another possible trigger.

EVENTS

Jot down in this column whenever something annoying, upsetting, or out of the ordinary happens. This could be anything from an argument to a tight deadline at work to an illness in the family. One word will probably be enough to remind you.

SYMPTOMS

This has to be a large column, unless you decide to use a similar form of shorthand to that for triggers. It is perhaps best to complete this column at the height of your headache, rather than wait for the next diary entry. This way you will not miss the less obvious symptoms; the symptom checklist below will also help here. You can copy it out on a separate sheet of paper and go down the list to 'check off' your symptoms.

Symptom checklist

- Warning signs
- Nausea
- Vomiting
- Diarrhoea
- Changes in vision

- Strange sensations
- One-sided pain
- Stabbing pain
- Throbbing pain
- Tight, 'pressure' pain
- Runny nose/streaming eyes
- Sensitivity to noise
- Sensitivity to light
- Other signs of nervous tension
    - fast heartbeat
    - sweating
    - 'butterflies' or churning stomach

MEDICATION

In this column, note down any medication that you take for your headache – which kind and how much.

Extracting the information

Sometimes it will be obvious from your diary when there is a link between something and your headaches. You may always get a migraine in the days before your period. Every time your shift changes you have a tension headache. It may also be possible to pick out the triggers that *don't* lead to headaches. In general, however, links have to be 'teased out'. The best way to do this is to plot a graph. A somewhat simplified example for a five week period is given overleaf. In this graph the average daily reading for both emotional and tension headache is used to plot each

Headaches

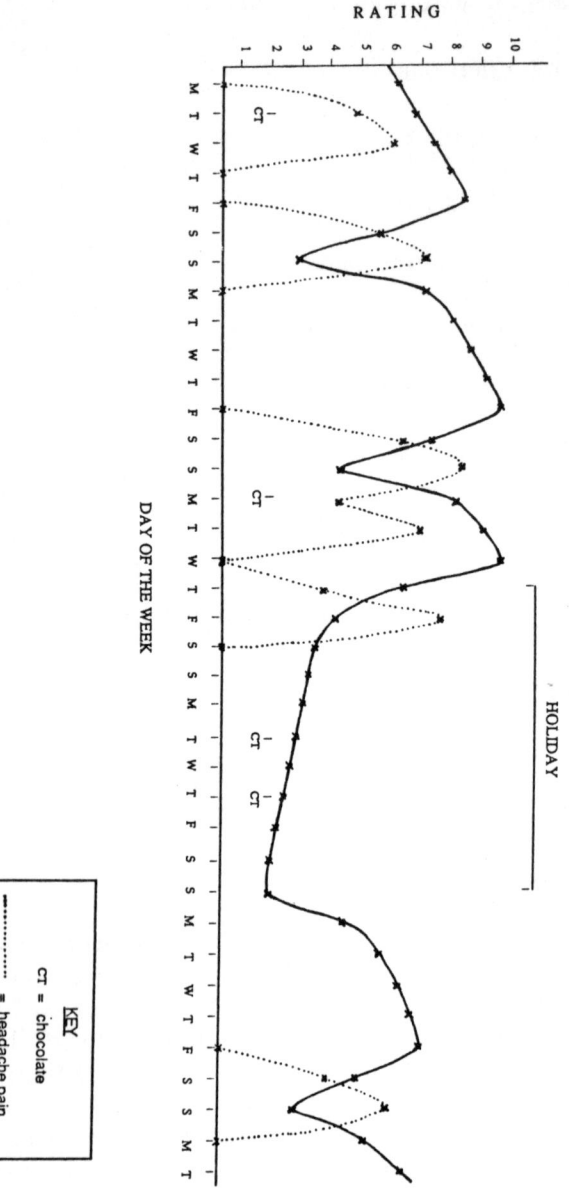

50

Recording your Headaches

point. Just add up the readings for breakfast, lunch, dinner and bedtime and divide by four, for each day. You can plot each individual reading if you like but this will make the graph even more complicated.

You can see that in this example headaches seem to happen when a period of emotional tension is *over* (a common pattern) – most often at the weekends. There is a definite link between tension and this person's headaches, although it is not the obvious one of more tension leading to more headaches. Chocolate does not seem to cause headaches on its own in this particular case. However, in combination with stress it does. This kind of finding is common, and is perhaps most marked in headaches that are linked to the menstrual cycle. Women often report that, for instance, when they are on holiday their menstrual headaches do not occur. Teasing out these interactions is not easy. If you are not a statistician or a computer whizz-kid then perhaps the best way is to look long and hard at your graphs. Come up with some educated guesses or hypotheses. Then test them out by looking to see if it is true over the whole period of your diary. Look particularly for stress adding to other factors and leading to a headache.

The next step is to use the information that you have gained. Cut out the factors that are triggering or worsening your headaches. Of course, this is easier in the case of food triggers than it is with, say, emotional tension. However, the following two chapters will give you many pointers on how to reduce such tension.

Remember to carry on keeping your headache diary over the period of any treatment that you try, so that you can keep tabs on how successful the treatment is. When using the diary for this purpose, it is probably best to record and plot both aspects of pain.

51

5. Learning How to Relax

'I don't need to learn how to relax'.
'I watch television to relax'.
'Things don't bother me that much really'.
'I'm quite happy so I can't be tense'.

These are some of the things that people say when I suggest to them that they learn relaxation techniques. They think that people who are tense and need to learn relaxation are somehow not normal – 'neurotic' or 'untogether'. This is simply not true. Everyone can benefit from learning how to relax. Even the most laid-back and apparently relaxed people have tensions that are over and above what they need – even when they are asleep. The word 'tension' means here physical tension, and not emotional tension, although the two are linked. Often, and perhaps more often than not, people do not realise that they are tense; they do not recognise their tension. Stop reading this book for a moment. How are you sitting? Are there any tensions in the muscles of your shoulders? Your neck? Back? Your hands? Are you clenching your jaw or frowning slightly? Most people find that they are much more tense than they need be. Part of the problem is that they don't realise it.

Learning how to relax is a skill like any other. You have to practise it. It does not come naturally. Watching television or reading a book is a form of relaxation in that it gives you a break from work. However, you can do these things while still being physically tense; most people do. The point is, because you do not in general recognise your tension, it does not occur to you to get rid of it. People develop the tension habit. A habit is something that you do continually and without thinking. It is difficult to stop. Tension is like this. Over your whole lifetime, because you have not learned ways to recognise and get rid of it, the tension has gradually built up. People get into a vicious circle: the more

Learning How to Relax

tense they are, the less they cope with life, the more tense they get. This refers to both emotional and physical tension, but it is probably the physical tension that makes it more difficult for you to cope. Even if life has been a bed of roses and you have always been happy, if you don't learn ways of getting rid of tension, it just builds up. Because the tension has built up so gradually, you forget what it is to be perfectly relaxed; as you get used to the tension, your baseline for being relaxed goes up and up. In other words, the level of muscular tension that you think of as 'relaxed' has gone up over the years as your tension has risen.

> 'How can I relax when I've got so much to do?'
> 'It sounds so time-consuming'.
> 'I can't relax when I've got bills to pay/when I've got deadlines at work'.

If you feel this way then you *definitely* need to learn to relax. People who feel that they should always be doing something are the ones who are most at risk from excessive tension. What you may not realise is that if you get rid of tension, you will feel so much better that you will be able to get on with life much more effectively. Not only will you not

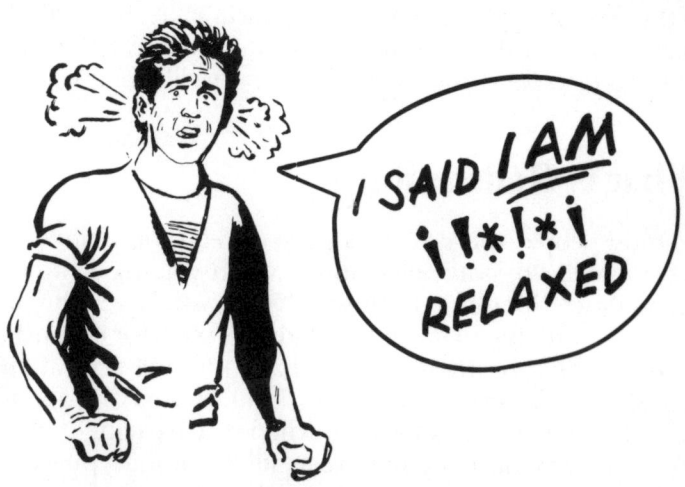

have so many headaches, but you will also find that you have more energy. Keeping muscles tense for much of your life uses up a lot of energy, so you get tired much more easily. Relaxing muscles releases energy for other purposes. You may also find that your attitude to life changes; when you are uptight it is difficult to get the most out of life. Physically relaxing does make you less uptight in general. You may find yourself on a positive cycle: the better you feel, the more you put in and get out of life, the better you feel. So the small investment in time for practising relaxation techniques will more than pay dividends in the long run. It is your health that is at stake.

'I can't relax with the children always around.'

There may be practical barriers to doing relaxation exercises, such as having the children to contend with. However, if you are committed enough, then you will find a way around those barriers. Suggestions are given in the section 'dealing with difficulties'. Commitment is all-important in learning relaxation. Because it is a skill like any other – like learning to drive, for instance – regular practice is essential. You have to work at breaking the tension habit, especially in everyday life. You have to gradually chip away at the tensions. The actual exercises will take about 20-30 minutes, twice a day. So only 40-60 minutes a day is the time you need to spend for your health and wellbeing.

What is Relaxation?

To most people, there are two kinds of relaxation: physical and mental. Physical relaxation is when you are lying or sitting down. Mental relaxation is when you have a break from life: listening to music, or reading a book for instance. If this is the case, then you can have physical relaxation without mental relaxation: you can still be worrying about the bills to pay or the jobs to do when you are lying down. You can also have mental relaxation without physical relaxation: playing sport, for instance, or dancing.

Learning How to Relax

However, neither lying down nor reading a book is necessarily true relaxation. Relaxation is the absence of tensions. You can be tense reading a book and lying down. So what actually are 'tensions' and 'relaxation'?

To find out what 'tensions' are you have to go back to Chapter 2 in which the nature of stress was discussed. If you remember, the stress reaction involves being continually anxious, uptight, aroused, or whatever word you would like to use. Being uptight or anxious means that your autonomic nervous system is turning itself up. This means, among other things, more adrenalin in your blood system. Adrenalin causes a number of changes in your body, including increases in muscle tension, faster heart beat, rapid shallow breathing, sweaty palms and so on. This is called *autonomic arousal* and is the direct opposite of relaxation. When you are highly aroused, as well as these physical changes, the adrenalin causes your mind to race as well. Your thoughts jump from one thing to another, probably from one worry to another, without solving anything. You experience this as being mentally uptight. So you can see that mental and physical tension are intimately linked.

The opposite of autonomic arousal is relaxation – when your autonomic nervous system turns itself down. This is the important thing as far as headaches are concerned. As discussed in Chapter 2, when the autonomic nervous system is wound up, causing muscle tensions and blood chemical changes, headaches become more likely. When you lower autonomic arousal, you find that not only do you physically relax but you also find that your mind races less. Like those few moments just before you drift off to sleep, you become mentally relaxed.

How can you prevent autonomic arousal? In many ways, but perhaps the most efficient is learning to relax your muscles. You cannot be aroused and have relaxed muscles at the same time – these states are at opposite ends of the spectrum. When you relax your muscles you are in effect turning down your autonomic nervous system. The rest of this chapter will suggest ways in which you can do this. First you must learn how to relax when everything is quiet and you are perfectly comfortable – relaxation exercises. When you are good at these you can start practising in more difficult situations and learning to relax in everyday life.

Relaxation Exercises

First, a word of warning. If you suffer any kind of medical condition then discuss with your doctor if learning to relax will complicate things. This is not to say that it is not safe; it is. However, the exercises may alter your body in ways that are usually beneficial – it can lower blood pressure, for instance – but this may complicate any treatment that you are receiving. For instance, if you are diabetic it may alter your insulin requirements.

In this book, two main types of relaxation exercises will be discussed. You can try them both for a fortnight and see which is better for you. Neither is superior for all people: it is a question of 'horses for courses'. The first type, called *progressive relaxation*, is the more well-researched technique, so try this first. You will know whether it is right for you within two weeks. If you start to feel it is working during this period then continue with it, because it has the advantage of teaching you how to recognise muscular tension.

Practise the relaxation exercises twice a day *and* whenever you feel a headache coming on. Do them in a quiet room that is not too bright. Choose a time when you are guaranteed no interruptions for at least half an hour. Don't practise immediately before going out or doing something to a deadline: you will just be distracted by thoughts about what you have to do. You can do the exercise lying on the floor or preferably in a comfortable armchair or recliner. The chair should support all your weight so that you do not have to tense any muscles while you are sitting. Make sure, in particular, that the small of your back, your legs, and your head and neck are properly supported; use little cushions if necessary. If you are on the floor have a small cushion under your neck and a smaller one under the back of your head – that way your neck will not be stretched. Loosen any tight clothing and remove glasses or contact lenses before you start.

Progressive relaxation

This kind of relaxation is of proven effectiveness. For the purposes of the exercises, the body is divided into a number of muscle groups – it doesn't matter how many. At first, probably the more the better. Your hand and forearm might be one muscle group, your upper arm another, and so on. The exercises involve first tensing and then relaxing each of these muscle groups in turn, while focusing your attention on the sensations involved. The reason for initially tensing the muscles is twofold. First, there appears to be a rebound effect, so that the muscles end up less tense than if you simply tried to relax them. Rather like a pendulum; if you want it to swing away from you, it is easier to pull it up towards you and then let it go than to try and push it away from you. You may also see the importance of suddenly letting the muscles relax, instead of gradually doing it.

The second reason for tensing the muscle group before you relax it is that you become more aware of what tension feels like, and how it differs from relaxation. That is why it is important for you to keep your mind on the sensations in your muscles (it also aids relaxation). You might think: 'I know that already!' or 'I only have to do that once to find that out'. However, knowing the difference between tension and relaxation is different from *being aware* of it in everyday life. You have to work at awareness – it is not something you get in a flash of inspiration. It has to sink in so that realising you are tense becomes second nature. Also, most people do *not* know true relaxation. What they think of as being 'relaxed' is probably just marginally less tense than they normally are.

The first stage then is to decide what the muscle groups are and to work out how you are going to tense them. It is probably best to start with at least the 15 different groups that are suggested below. However, you can increase the number if you want to, for instance, by separating the hands and forearm or the calves and the feet. You may find that by doing this you can relax more successfully.

The important thing when you are deciding on tensing methods is that you have to be able to *feel* the tension. The ones suggested here are generally good from this point of view, but if you cannot feel the tension then try and work out an alternative. The other important thing to remember is that you have to be able to tense a particular group of muscles without tensing muscles in other groups. If you have just relaxed the muscles in your hand and forearm, for instance, and you are tensing the muscles in your upper arm, then you want to keep the muscles in your hand and forearm completely relaxed while you are doing so. Otherwise you spoil the whole point of the exercise, which is to relax each muscle group in turn until your whole body is relaxed.

Tensing muscle groups

Try tensing each of these muscle groups using the methods suggested before you try the actual relaxation technique. Tense the muscles as hard as you can and decide which strategies are best for you. Do this when you are seated or lying down, as you would be when you practise the actual exercise.

> *Hand and forearm:* try clenching your fist as tightly as you can. If you can't feel your forearm muscles, then try doing the same but pushing your fist upwards.
> *Upper arm:* try making the two main muscles in your upper arm as hard as you can – the one that runs along the front (biceps) and the one that runs along the back (triceps). If this does not work then try pressing your elbow down on to the chair or floor; some people prefer

pressing their elbow downwards and inwards at the same time.
Foot and lower leg: curling your toes tightly will tense your foot. You can tense your calves either by pointing your foot away from you and inwards at the same time, or towards your head. Do this while tensing your foot. Some people prefer just making their calves as hard as they can.
Upper leg and buttocks: try making your thighs and buttocks rock solid. Alternatively, lift your whole leg up an inch or two from the floor or chair. Make sure you can feel the tension in the whole upper leg and buttocks.

Do the above first with the right and then the left arm and leg.

Stomach: the best strategy is to make your stomach as hard as you can, as if someone were going to hit you there. If you cannot feel the tension, then try arching your back at the same time. If you do this, feel the tension also in your lower back. Some people like to tense the lower back separately.
Back, chest and shoulders: take a deep breath and while you are doing so try and make your shoulder blades meet. Notice the tension all over the back, your chest and probably your shoulders (the last does not matter too much since there is a separate exercise for the shoulders). In the exercise, you let go the breath when you release the tension.
Shoulders: try to make your shoulders touch your ears (don't expect to do so!). If this is not effective, try pushing your shoulders forward at the same time.
Neck: try 'counterpoising' the muscles at the back of your neck with the muscles at the front of your neck. That is, tense both as hard as you can. If you cannot feel the tension all the way around, try pushing your head back against the chair or floor. Alternatively, if you are lying down, lift your head an inch or two from the floor.
Lower face and jaw: clench your teeth together as hard as

possible, while at the same time pulling the corners of your mouth outwards or downwards. If you cannot feel the tension in your jaw, then try sticking your bottom jaw outwards and upwards as far as it will go.
Upper face: screw up your face as tightly as you can – tense your nose, mouth, and eyes all together. Make sure your jaw stays relaxed.
Forehead: you can either raise your eyebrows as high as possible, or frown as deeply as you can. Try and feel the tension all around your head.

As you may have noticed, the exercises concentrate particularly around the head, neck and shoulders. This is because these muscles are involved in many headaches of both the tension and migraine kind. Probably the best order of the exercises is the one in the list above, gradually working up the body and finishing with the head. In which case the order would be: right hand and lower arm, right upper arm, left hand and lower arm, left upper arm, right foot and lower leg, right upper leg and buttocks, left foot and lower leg, left upper leg and buttocks, stomach, (possibly lower back), back and chest, shoulders, neck, jaw, face, and lastly forehead. That is at least 15 muscle groups; the order that you do them in is, however, entirely up to you. Make sure that the order you do them in enables you to keep the previous muscle group relaxed while you are tensing the next.

Doing the exercises

You should now know what muscle groups you are going to use and how you are going to tense them. You can now practise the relaxation exercises. Use one of the following methods:

> *Memorise the exercise yourself.* This is perhaps the best way, so that you can be entirely self-dependent. You can also do the exercises at your own pace, the way you are

Learning How to Relax

feeling at the moment. Once you know the tensing methods and the order in which to relax the muscle groups then all you really have to remember is: first, when you release the tension do it suddenly, and second, try to keep your mind on the sensations in your muscles.

Make a tape-recording of the instructions so that you can do the exercises listening to it. Some suggestions for the wording of the instructions are given below. Keep your voice sounding fairly monotonous and talk at a 'plodding' pace, except when the muscles are being tensed – sound tense, talk more quickly. Elsewhere, don't try and sound 'relaxing' because on tape it will probably sound hilarious. Make a few recordings and use the best. A useful hint is actually to do the exercises (as far as possible!) when you are recording – that way you will get the timing right, and will use the correct kind of words for your sensations. Lastly, don't talk too much, it can be distracting.

Get another person involved, and you can give each other the relaxation instructions. Many people would like to benefit from learning how to relax – they need not suffer from headaches. The hints for the tape-recording are equally relevant to this method.

The exercises involve tensing a muscle group for perhaps five or six seconds, and then letting go of the tension all at once. You then carry on relaxing the muscle group for 20 to 30 seconds. The exact timing is not important but give enough time to focus your attention on the feelings in your muscles, and above all *don't rush*. It is best to breathe in just before tensing the muscles, hold your breath during, and release it when you release the tension. Repeat this tension-relaxation cycle at least twice with each muscle group when you first start learning the exercises. You will find that the muscles will be more relaxed after the second tensing than the first. It doesn't matter how many times you tense and relax a muscle group – keep doing it until you feel it is completely relaxed. Remember to leave at least 20

Headaches

seconds for the relaxation phases. Once you have achieved relaxation in the muscle group then you can move on to the next. Do the same with that muscle group, while keeping the first muscles completely relaxed. And so on. When you have finished all the muscle groups, stay in the relaxed state for a few minutes to enjoy the sensations. Then *slowly* bring yourself back to reality – some hints on this are given below.

Relaxation instructions

The following paragraph will give you an idea of the kind of words and descriptions that may be used for relaxation instructions. There is, however, no substitute for your own words. It can be very distracting, for instance, if, when you are relaxing some muscles, the instructions are saying '. . . feel the muscles unwind . . . smooth out . . .' when the muscles don't feel that way at all! I will give you the beginning of the exercise, to give you an idea of a good way of starting; the tensing and relaxing of one muscle group; and the ending. These are just suggestions so please do not take them as the 'right' way to do it. The 'right' way is what feels best for you.

Beginning, and tensing and relaxing one muscle group

> Make sure you are sitting comfortably . . . just sit there for a few moments to enjoy the calm and stillness that is around you . . . when you are ready feel your eyelids close . . . concentrate on your breathing for a few moments . . . feel the cool air come in through your nostrils . . . down into your lungs . . . and feel the warm air come out . . . let your breathing slow down . . . breathe right down into your lungs . . . feel your tummy rise and fall with each breath . . . cool air in . . . warm air out . . . just concentrate like that for a few moments . . . When you are ready, bring your attention on to the muscles of your right hand and forearm. When I say, I want you to tense these as hard as you can by forming a tight fist and pointing your fist upwards . . . ready? *Now* . . .

feel the muscles pulling, feel them tight, hard . . . hold it . . . and *relax* . . . let go of the tension . . . just let it drift off . . . feel the muscles unwind . . . notice the difference between the tension and the relaxation . . . just let the muscles smooth out . . . loosen up . . . as the warm relaxation spreads into the muscles of your hand and forearm . . . just let that last bit of tension drift off . . . now, I want you to shift your attention on to the muscles of your right upper arm. In a moment, I will ask you to tense those muscles by pressing your elbow down onto the chair and inwards at the same time. Do this while keeping the muscles of your lower arm and hand completely relaxed. Ready? *Now* . . .

and so on.

Ending

Just sit there for a few minutes enjoying the feelings of warm relaxation . . . let the last bit of tension drift off . . . from your arms . . . your legs . . . feel your forehead smooth out . . . unwind . . . as you relax more and deeply . . . let your head feel heavy and relaxed . . . your arms feel heavy and relaxed . . . feel yourself sinking as your whole body basks in the feeling of warm relaxation . . . enjoy these relaxed feelings for a few moments more . . .

When you are ready, I am going to bring you back to the here and now . . . I am going to count slowly backwards from five to one . . . when I say five, I want you to start moving your fingers; when I say four, start moving your arms as well; three, your toes; on two, move your legs around; and on one, I want you to open your eyes and have a look around you . . . and you will feel completely relaxed and refreshed and ready to face the world. Ready? Five . . . just wiggle your fingers slowly . . . feel them come back to life, the blood flowing through them . . . four . . .

and so on, counting backwards slowly.

Notice that in these instructions the emphasis is on the *sensations* in the muscles, so that the difference between tension and relaxation is highlighted. Words such as 'pulling', 'tight', 'bunching', 'hard', and so on are good for the tensing phase. Words such as 'unwind', 'smooth out', 'drift off', 'loosen', 'limp', and so on are good for the relaxation phase. Calling attention to feelings of warmth and heaviness is also very good for general relaxation (provided you can feel these – some people feel light, for instance). Indeed, this is the basis for the other form of relaxation in this book, autogenic relaxation. If you do the exercises on your own, try saying some of the phrases in your head – particularly the word 'relax' as you let go of the tension.

Lastly, make sure you are breathing in a relaxed manner. This means slowly but easily, and breathing so that your tummy moves up and down, not your chest. Chest breathing comes with autonomic arousal, and you want to achieve the opposite. Relaxed breathing will mean deeper relaxation.

Dealing with problems

'I'm never on my own long enough to practise.' This can be a real problem, especially if you have children. Although it is best to practise twice a day, if you can manage only once a day then you will still benefit enormously. Because you have to do it regularly, finding a babysitter may well be impossible. Try getting the help of a neighbour, particularly one who also wants to learn to relax. Persuade her of the benefits! If she also has children, you can take turns with the kids. Or explain to the children that you want some time on your own – they may be willing to co-operate from a younger age than you would expect!

'I can't seem to fully relax.' Don't worry, it will come in the end. Many people take weeks of regular practising before they can relax properly. Like any skill, practice makes perfect. Remember, it has taken you years and years to build up the tension habit so it's not going to be easy to break it. The main thing is not to force it; just let the relaxation happen in its own good time. The more you worry about not relaxing, the less relaxed you will be!

'I get strange feelings when I'm relaxing.' These are common and no two people feel exactly the same way when they relax. You may feel that you are floating away, or falling, or sinking. You may feel that you are paralysed. Some people even start to feel worried or anxious. This is probably because the state of relaxation is an entirely new experience for them. Just carry on practising and these worries will pass. Sometimes, people fear that they will lose control over what happens, and that is why relaxation is frightening to them. The only way to get over these fears is to carry on practising so that your body learns that there is nothing to be afraid of. If the fears are so strong that it means that you cannot relax, then just concentrate on your breathing for 10 or 20 minutes. Once you have practised this a few times and are used to it, introduce concentrating on the feelings in your muscles. Practise this until it feels safe. Then perhaps introduce tensing and relaxing one muscle group only. Keep practising until it feels OK. Then try two muscle groups, and so on until you are able to do the whole exercise.

'I get pins and needles.' Make sure your clothing is loose enough and the room is warm. Make sure also that the chair that you are using is supporting the whole of your body. If it is still a problem, keep practising and it may go away. Pins and needles are due to poor blood circulation, and the more you relax the better your circulation should be; if your muscles are tense the blood does not flow very well. If all fails and you find the pins and needles too distracting (they are not harmful in themselves) then try autogenic relaxation, which, incidentally, can improve your circulation. However, if you have low blood pressure then go to your doctor for advice.

'I get cramps when I try tensing my muscles.' Again, this is quite common, particularly in the legs and toes. In which case, try tensing not quite so hard. Part of the reason that you may get cramps is that you rarely use some of these muscles, in which case this problem should ease with

practice. It may also be a sign that these muscles are particularly tense, so bear with it.

'I get fits of giggles.' Another common problem. If you are using a tape or if you are doing the exercises with a companion and you find the instructions funny, change them. If it is the situation or the voice that you find funny then that will pass with familiarity. So keep practising. If you have no idea why you giggle, then don't concern yourself with it, just let it pass. It will. Often people giggle as a means of releasing tension, so just get it out of your system.

'I keep getting distracted by noises and things.' No matter where the room is, there will always be noises. Try to accept them and just let them drift in one ear and out the other. Don't get uptight about all the distractions because you will only be creating more tensions for yourself. If you do get distracted, simply bring your mind back to the sensations in your muscles. The better you get at relaxing, the less noises will be a problem.

'My mind keeps wandering.' Treat this in the same way as the outside distractions. Don't worry and just gently bring your attention back to your muscles. If your mind races, then that is a sign of autonomic arousal and will lessen as you get better at relaxing.

'I keep falling asleep.' Try not to, because then you will not be reaping all of the benefits from the exercises. You can still sleep with tense muscles. You will find that your mind starts to wander just before nodding off; if you can keep your attention focused on the feelings in your muscles this should be less of a problem. By the way, if you have trouble sleeping, then these relaxation techniques can be a very effective way of getting off to sleep. And because your muscles are more relaxed, you also sleep more deeply.

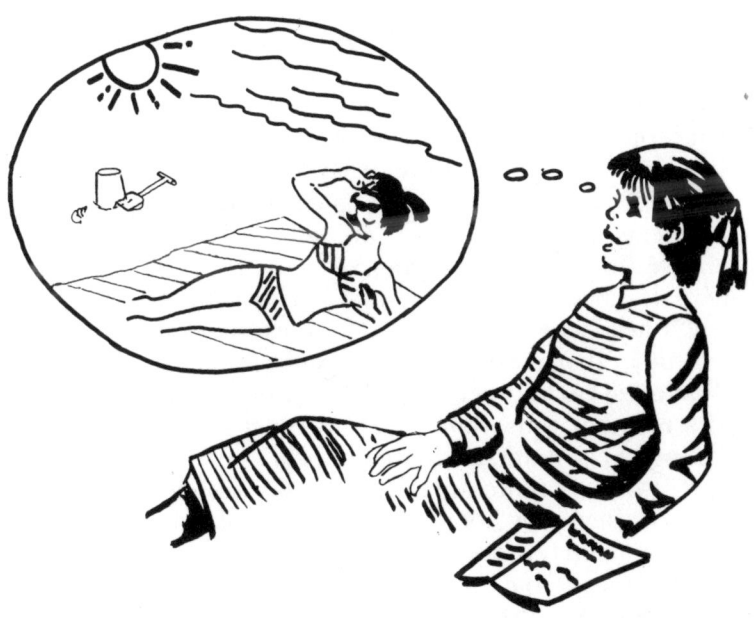

Autogenic relaxation

These exercises are much simpler than progressive relaxation but can achieve the same effect. The main disadvantage is that you do not specifically learn to recognise muscle tension, although people often find that regular experience of deep relaxation naturally raises their awareness of tension in their everyday lives. Autogenic relaxation is a bit more like meditation in that you have to concentrate on a series of relaxing phrases that you say to yourself in your head. You can make similar arrangements to the progressive relaxation exercises, as well as trying to remember them – making a tape, or involving somebody else – but in this case the exercises will be much more effective if you do them yourself.

Autogenic exercises were developed for people to do them on their own; the word 'autogenic' means 'coming from within'. The phrases that you have to remember are very simple. They are to do with your body feeling warm and heavy, which as you know often happens when you are relaxed. Curiously, just saying these things and concentrating on your body allows your body to relax. It is a kind of suggestion, and so is sometimes called *auto-suggestion* because you have to say the phrases to yourself.

Where you practise, how you prepare yourself, and problems that may occur are all similar to those in progressive relaxation so there is no point repeating them here. It is best to practise at least twice a day and when you feel a headache coming on. These exercises take slightly less time than progressive relaxation, but ideally they should still last between 15 and 20 minutes. The main thing to remember with these exercises is *not to force them*. Any feelings or sensations that come will come in their own time. Don't *try* to do anything. If your muscles don't feel warm or heavy try not to concern yourself – worrying will stop you from relaxing. People often feel very little but that doesn't mean that nothing is happening – measurable decreases in autonomic arousal can still occur. Keep practising and you will find that you feel more and more relaxed as your skill improves.

The exercises

Start in the same way as with the progressive relaxation, by closing your eyes and concentrating on your breathing. Then say to yourself in your head (that is, without actually speaking): '*I am feeling calm and relaxed*'. Some people prefer: '*I am feeling relaxed and at peace with myself*'. Or, if you find it grates because you don't feel that way, try just saying single words: '*calm*', '*relax*', '*peace*', or anything similar. This first stage of the exercise is just to prepare you and get you in the right frame of mind, so the exact phrases are not important. Whatever you do say to yourself, say it calmly and fairly slowly. Then let the words sink in for a while, and then repeat the phrase. Do this for as many times as you wish, at least four. All the while let your mind stay with your breathing.

When you are ready, move your attention on to your right arm and say to yourself, *'my right arm is heavy'*. Let the words sink in. Feel the arm's weight. Your arm *is* heavy; quite a few pounds. View it as though it were not part of your body. Visualise your arm lying heavily on the armrest or floor. Then repeat the phrase. Carry on passively observing your arm's heaviness. Repeat the phrase at least four times, leaving a decent gap in between. Then move on to your right leg, and do the same. Then your left leg, left arm, back, shoulders, neck, and lastly head. Above all, don't rush and don't force it. Keep a passive, observing attitude.

The next stage of the exercise is to focus on feelings of warmth. So, when you are ready, move your attention on to your right arm again and say to yourself, *'my right arm is warm'*. Let yourself feel the warmth. Your arm *is* warm; the blood flowing through it is warm. Picture its warmth. If you like, imagine the feeling of the summer sun warming the skin on your arm. Let the feeling of warmth spread. Repeat the phrase and again let the words sink in. Do this at least four times, more if you wish. Enjoy those feelings of warmth. Move on to your right leg when you are ready, then your left leg, and so on, leaving out your head this time. Remain a passive observer: your body is warm.

For the last few minutes keep your attention on your forehead. Say to yourself: *'my forehead is cool'* and imagine your forehead feeling pleasantly cool. This will relax it even further; headache sufferers often have trouble relaxing their forehead. Then enjoy the relaxed feelings of warmth and heaviness, just as you did in the progressive relaxation exercises, and bring yourself back to reality in the same way. If you like, before you start to count backwards, say to yourself a few times, *'I am refreshed and ready to face the world'*, or something similar. And you will be!

Shortening the exercises

After a few weeks of practising twice a day, you should find that you become more and more relaxed during the exercises. Continue until you go for a whole week without further improvement or until you feel that you can relax *completely*. Then – and then only – you can start shortening the exercises. Shorten them in stages, and at each stage continue until you again feel that you can reach total relaxation using the shorter method.

Progressive relaxation
First, you can try just tensing and relaxing each muscle group once only. Shorten or miss out concentrating on your breathing at the beginning. Continue this for a few weeks, still practising twice a day. When this makes you just as relaxed as tensing each muscle group twice, you can start combining the groups. Try:

- your right hand, lower arm and upper right arm together. Just combine the tensing strategies.
- same with your left arm.
- your right foot, lower leg, and upper leg together.
- same with your left leg.
- your tummy together with your chest and back.
- your neck.
- combine all three facial strategies, although you may like to keep the forehead one separate.

It is particularly important to remember to breathe in just before the tensing, hold the breath during, and to release it with the word 'relax' while using these shorter techniques.

This list is just a suggestion, and indeed you can combine the muscle groups in any way that you feel is effective. Don't worry about how it must look! When these methods produce total relaxation, you can combine the muscle groups even further: both legs together, and both arms together. It is probably best to keep the others separate. The whole exercise using these strategies should take little more than ten minutes, but *never* rush. At each stage make sure that you can get completely relaxed.

In the last stage, you can leave out the tensing altogether. By this time your body will be relaxing well when you want it to, and the relaxation will be associated with the word 'relax' together with letting the breath out. So try the whole exercise but instead of actually tensing the muscle groups just notice the tension that is already there. Do this while holding your breath; then in your head say the word 'relax' while letting the breath out, and see if the tension drifts off. Let your muscles unwind in the same way as after you have deliberately tensed them. Eventually you will be able to relax completely just using the word 'relax' and the breath out.

Autogenic relaxation

Shortening the autogenic exercises is a simpler affair, but depends more on your good judgement as to what you can cut out, while still keeping the exercise as effective. The options are:

> Fewer repetitions of each phrase. As you get better at relaxing, you will find that you relax more quickly so that the third and fourth repetitions of each phrase may be unnecessary.
> Shorten or leave out the concentration on breathing.
> Leave out completely either the 'heavy' stage or the 'warming' stage: many people find one of these clearly superior.
> Combine the 'heavy' and 'warm' phrases: for instance, 'My right arm is warm and heavy'.

Whichever you choose, remember that you should never rush. The passive, waiting frame of mind is central to autogenic relaxation. Whatever will come, will come.

Applying Relaxation Skills to 'Real Life'

Many people find that there are real benefits in practising relaxation skills even if they don't consciously apply them to real life. You may find that your headaches are reduced in both intensity and frequency. The benefits probably occur through three processes. First, the two 'doses' of relaxation a day will prevent tension from building up. Second, doing the exercises to stop a headache from developing or reducing its intensity will not only reduce headaches but also reduce the stress resulting from having a headache. And third, particularly with progressive relaxation, you may find yourself naturally becoming more aware of your tension. There are other ways of making even more of your relaxation skills.

To speed up the process of becoming totally aware of your tension, throughout the day at frequent times stop and 'take stock'. If you are managing to keep a headache diary, you will be used to rating your emotional tension. Well, every time you stop, try mentally rating your *physical* tension as well. In your head, go over your whole body – muscle group by muscle group – and note how tense they are. This should take less than a minute and can be done anywhere. You may like to note down your overall rating (from one to ten) in your diary to keep tabs on how well you are doing. Try to 'take stock' in this way as often as possible, at least every hour.

Whenever you can, try relaxing your whole body for a minute or two. You will get better at these 'quick' relaxations as you improve with practising at home. Indeed, as you shorten the exercises you may find that you can fit one or two full relaxations in during your working day. Otherwise, try a 'quick' relaxation as often as possible. You can do this in a number of ways. You can concentrate on your breathing for a minute or two. You can mentally go over your whole body and relax each muscle group in turn.

In fact, when you become adept at relaxing you can do this whenever you 'take stock'. You can use your best autogenic phrases. Or, if you use progressive relaxation, you can say the word 'relax' after holding a breath, so that the tension evaporates as you let the breath out – just as you do during the exercises proper. All of these 'quick' relaxations can be done with your eyes open or closed, so that they can easily be fitted in during the day – and nobody need notice. Do them especially around the time of any stressful event.

The more you stop and practise 'taking stock' and 'quick' relaxations, the more benefits will be felt. If you do the relaxation exercises when you feel a headache coming on, so that it is aborted or reduced in intensity, this means that you are also avoiding the stress of the headache itself. These things, and the doses of deep relaxation at home, will ensure that your autonomic arousal level will be kept as low as possible throughout the day. It will make you feel a more relaxed person. However, many things will still upset you even though you do your best to stop them making you tense. Read through Chapter 6 to get some ideas about how to reduce these kind of life stresses.

Cutting out stimulants

Have you ever noticed an adrenalin 'rush' when you have to do important work to a deadline, or play an important sports game? That is the extra energy that the adrenalin temporarily gives you when your levels of autonomic arousal are high. Stimulants work by getting your autonomic nervous system to turn itself up in exactly the same way. As you may remember, this is the exact *opposite* of what you are trying to achieve with relaxation techniques. To make matters worse, when you are 'hyped-up' on a stimulant, you tend to rush around trying to fit too much in, you get irritable, you can't sleep properly – all of which increase stress levels. Stress increases autonomic arousal, and before you know it you are caught in a vicious circle. It becomes obvious, then, that people who suffer from stress-related problems would do well to avoid *all* stimulants.

Caffeine

This is a stimulant that is very difficult to avoid. Apart from being in tea and coffee, caffeine is in a wide range of soft drinks and medications. You may think that it is a relatively weak or harmless substance. You would be wrong. The amount of caffeine in only two cups of coffee can increase your blood levels of adrenalin – a sure sign of autonomic arousal – by about three times. And it takes your body up to ten hours just to get rid of half of it. As you can see, caffeine is both a powerful and long-lasting stimulant.

Caffeine increases headaches in a number of ways. First, like all stimulants, it increases autonomic arousal so making headaches more likely. Second, being 'hyped-up' means that you act in a way that increases your stress levels. Third, as discussed in Chapter 3, caffeine can cause *rebound* headaches. Caffeine constricts your blood vessels so that when you do without it your blood vessels swell up, sometimes past their normal size – causing a headache. People can become addicted to caffeine in this way. They have to take it to avoid these headaches, but the more caffeine they take the more likely the rebound headaches are. People can also become *psychologically* addicted to caffeine. After the initial 'rush', they become much less efficient, more irritable, and find it more difficult to concentrate. This is because that extra energy did not come from nowhere! So they take more caffeine to pep them up. And so on.

It is obvious that if you are learning to relax it is *essential* that you avoid caffeine. Even one cup of coffee a day can cause problems! People are sensitive to caffeine to varying extents, but the effects on the body are such that it will act against all you are trying to achieve with the relaxation exercises. You may find that trying to do without caffeine leads to more headaches. These will be rebound headaches, and will only be temporary. They can be helped by using relaxation and painkillers and by cutting down on your caffeine consumption *gradually* over a period of a month. Don't be tempted to ask the doctor for other drugs that work by shrinking the blood vessels – ergotamine for instance; and don't use alcohol to help with the pain – this also dilates blood vessels. It may be a question of putting up with extra headaches in the short term to have fewer and be more healthy in the long term.

What are the things to avoid if you decide to give up caffeine? Tea and coffee are the obvious culprits. Decaffeinated teas and coffee are fine, as are herb teas such as chamomile. Some so-called herb teas do contain caffeine, however, so do look on the label and see if ordinary tea is an ingredient. Chocolate and cocoa also contain caffeine and similar substances. Cola drinks of all kinds are to be avoided for the same reason. Lastly, many medications for headache – both prescribed and non-prescribed – contain caffeine, as do some medicines for other problems. Ask your doctor or chemist if they do – but *don't* withdraw from any prescribed medication without your doctor's advice.

Other stimulants

Adrenalin and adrenalin-like substances are to be found in many medications. These are to be avoided for similar reasons to caffeine, although rebound headaches are not a danger. Nevertheless, these chemicals are very effective at raising your autonomic arousal levels, since adrenalin is part of your body's way of doing this. Adrenalin, also known as epinephrine, is an active ingredient in some asthma inhalers. Medicines for colds and 'flu, blocked noses, sinus problems, and so on, often contain adrenalin-like chemicals such as ephedrine. So do some medications for asthma and general allergies, and also weight-reducing tablets. Again, ask your chemist or doctor if any of these medications that you are taking contain adrenalin-like substances. If they are not being prescribed by your doctor, then withdraw those that do. If they are, get together with your doctor and see if anything else will do.

Tobacco is another stimulant you would do well to cut out for your headaches' sake. This is dealt with in Chapter 7.

You may be pleasantly surprised at the effects of cutting out stimulants. Apart from any effects on headaches, you may find yourself being calmer, more even-tempered, and having more energy. Some people find that they are less anxious or depressed. You will sleep better. These changes will also have positive 'knock on' effects, so that your life becomes less stressful in general. For instance, in the long run your relationships or standard of work might improve. Other ways of reducing stress in your everyday life are discussed in the next chapter.

Does Learning to Relax Reduce Headaches?

There have been many scientific studies to show that learning relaxation exercises greatly eases headaches in many cases. On average, people's headaches are halved in number. Some people become symptom-free; some don't benefit at all; but most are somewhere in between. Used in conjunction with dietary changes you have a good chance of reducing your headaches considerably. These are some of the things that headache sufferers have said to me after learning relaxation techniques:

Migraine sufferers:

> 'I have less headaches now, and most are less severe ... I think I have benefited by realising how much tension can be built up most days, and training myself to relax before the critical point is reached'.

'My headaches occur less often now. In general, I feel that I am a much more relaxed person in myself. I notice that I seem to be able to tackle, and only think about, one chore at a time without getting into a state and wondering to myself: "How am I going to get all this done by 4 o'clock?" and so on.'

'My headaches are less frequent now, and when I have a headache, instead of fighting it and making it worse I am now more relaxed, which alleviates it.'

Tension headache sufferers:

'I don't seem to get any headaches at all now. It made me realise that I had it in me to help myself and control my stress, tension, or whatever, because I definitely think this was the reason for the headaches in the first place. I used to worry about little things that did not matter and let things build up to a pitch where I would get a massive headache.'

'I have fewer headaches now ... I can recognise when I am tense more easily now, often before it's progressed as far as a headache.'

'My headaches are less intense and of shorter duration. I now feel a little in control when I have a headache. I know it will not interfere in my life like it did before. I can still continue to do things, knowing that in a couple of hours it will be gone.'

6. Your Lifestyle and Your Headaches

How Lifestyle Can Affect Headaches

People create their own stress. Stress isn't a thing that floats around waiting to inflict itself upon you. As Chapter 2 explained, stress is your reaction to situations, not the situations themselves. You make the stress for yourself. And stress begets stress: tense people rush around, find it difficult to concentrate, make poor decisions, sleep badly, and so on – all of which create more stress. Which causes more headaches. The relaxation exercises in the previous chapter will teach you how to lower your general levels of tension. At the same time, however, the pressure of stressful events will be forcing your levels of tension up. So it is important to learn also how to reduce the stress in your life, and how to deal with stressful situations. This chapter will give you some suggestions for this.

Changing your lifestyle

Feeling uptight, tense, anxious, under pressure, on edge – all these are part of the stress reaction. Why do we get these feelings?

> 'It's my job. It puts me under pressure.'
> 'I never get a minute of peace.'
> 'The children won't let me alone.'
> 'There's never enough time to fit everything in.'
> 'We're always arguing.'

People say that they get these feelings because of what happens to them – the pressurised job, the demanding children, the argumentative husband. They would say that all of these things are not under their control. So it is impossible to reduce stress levels without some drastic action, such as leaving their job or divorcing their husband. This, of course, may be true, but is usually only part of the story. Often something *can* be done, but for one reason or another isn't. The underlying reasons are often emotional rather than practical. Change might be frightening to you. You might be afraid of putting your needs first in case you are rejected. The standards that you set for yourself may be too high.

Take a long hard look at your life and see what needs to be changed to reduce your stress levels. Think: 'If that were a friend's life and they had too much stress, what would I advise them to change?' The best way of making changes is to use *problem solving* methods –these are discussed later in this chapter. But to make these changes, you often have to overcome emotional barriers: feeling that you should put everyone's needs before your own, feeling that it would be a disaster if you fail, feeling that you would be disliked if you stood up for yourself. So to make these changes you need to take charge of your own life. These difficulties are covered later in this chapter in the discussions on assertiveness and emotional problems. Towards the end of this chapter are some concrete suggestions on how most people should change their lifestyle if they are to overcome their headaches. The three main guidelines are: sleep better, take more exercise, and change your attitude to your headaches.

Reducing stress

The first step in learning how to reduce your stress levels is noticing how you are feeling and what your body is doing. If you do relaxation regularly you will become much more aware when you are becoming physically tense. Your

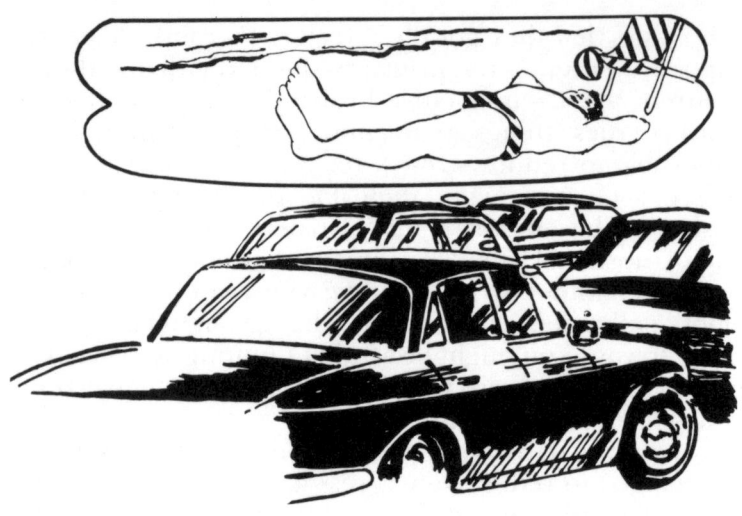

awareness will improve further if you are also frequently stopping and 'taking stock' in the way that was suggested in the last chapter. Physical tension is always a sure sign of being stressed.

Try also to stop what you are doing at regular intervals during the day to see how *emotionally* tense you are. How are you feeling? Under pressure? A sense of urgency? Worrying about the consequences of failure? The more you become aware of your physical and emotional state the more you can do about it. You can then use stress as a *cue* for anti-stress measures. Among the most powerful of these are, of course, relaxation techniques. So, at frequent times during the day, stop, note your physical and emotional state, and do something about it.

Perhaps the simplest strategy for reducing stress is detachment. Take time out. Switch off for a few minutes. Imagine a relaxing, pleasant scene – lying on the beach in the warm sun, for instance. You can practise detachment at tea breaks at work. Or when you need to wait in a queue or traffic jam, or any other 'boring' situation. Combine 'detachments' with the 'quick relaxations' mentioned in the previous chapter.

If you are at home during the day, or if you can do so at work, try to get a ten-minute break every two hours. Remember, your health is more important than housework or the company profits. You don't need to feel guilty, because in the long run you will be able to perform much better. Someone who is relaxed and headache-free is much more of an asset than someone who has difficulty in coping and often has to contend with a thumping headache.

Problem solving

You will get better and better at recognising whenever you are getting worked up or stressed. The next stage is to stop and consider where the emotional tension is coming from: what situation are you reacting to? People often take work tensions home with them, or home tensions to work. Analyse why you are uptight –and then do something about it. Think of the situation as a problem. The best way to do this is to phrase it: 'I need to. . .' Be specific. That will give you something concrete to aim for. Thinking of your needs might seem selfish but if it reduces stress levels, it will reduce your headaches and enable you to give much more to others in the long run. The quotes from people who were feeling stressed given at the beginning of this chapter might be rephrased as follows:

> *'It's my job. It puts me under pressure'* might become: 'I need to reduce the amount of work I do by at least one third'.
> *'I never get a minute of peace'* might become: 'I need to have at least one hour a day to myself'.
> *'We're always arguing'* might become: 'I need to be in a relationship where there are no resentments and everything is above board'.

Once you have a specific goal in mind, you can then set about achieving that goal – *solving the problem*. The best way of doing this is to 'brainstorm' as many solutions as you can think of – no matter how ridiculous, far-out, or frightening they may seem. Enlist the help of a close friend. Get as many ideas as possible, and get them down on paper. For instance, 'I need to reduce the amount of work I do by at least one third' might bring out the following ideas:

- do nothing;
- leave my job;
- change my job but stay with the same company;
- go part-time;
- ask my boss to give me less work;
- delegate more;
- job-share;
- refuse to do overtime;
- contact my union.

You now have a whole list of practical changes that you can make to solve your problem. The next stage is to list their 'pros' and 'cons': their advantages and disadvantages. The 'cons' of many of the options in this example will be to do with reduced pay or being difficult to achieve. The 'pros' would be to do with how much your work would be reduced and any other benefits. For instance, the 'pros' of 'ask my boss to give me less work' might be:

> 'It will reduce my work, but not by a third. I would feel better about myself because I have made my needs known. My boss might think more of me for the same reason. Other people

might be encouraged to do the same and we might get more staff. The quality of my work might go up because I would be less rushed'.

Whereas the 'cons' might be:

'My boss might think less of me and so it might damage the chances of promotion. I would be scared of doing it'.

Often you can think of ways to avoid some of the 'cons', like suggesting to your boss that the quality of your work will improve. The next stage is to decide between your options. Some people like to give scores according to how good the 'pros' are and how bad the 'cons' are. You can rate each advantage and each disadvantage out of ten. The five benefits for 'ask my boss to give me less work' might rate a score of 28 when added together, and the two disadvantages 12. Another option may have different 'pros' and 'cons' scores. Having gone through your list, you can then choose the option that gives you the best overall difference. Other people prefer just to read through their list and gradually whittle it down by rejecting the solutions in which the 'cons' are too high. Either way, you will arrive at a practical way of approaching your problem. (You may decide to put more than one of the options into action.) Then put the plan into action and see what happens. If unsuccessful, try the next best option.

You may be worried about making major decisions using what may seem to be little more than a parlour game. However, it is important that you see life stresses as problems to be solved and not just life being rotten to you. Solving problems in this way makes sure you take into account *all* the options. It means that you take a decision on a rational basis and that you take control. And perhaps most importantly, it means that your needs are taken into account. If you don't meet your needs – especially for time and space for yourself – then this will be a continual source of stress.

Headaches

Asserting yourself

Many of the options that you may come up with when you are solving your stress problems will involve asserting yourself, which means *making your needs known*. It does *not* mean being selfish or aggressive, because it does not mean that you impose your needs on other people. By ensuring your needs are met as far as possible you will be under less stress, so you will feel stronger and have fewer headaches, enabling you to give more to others. People who don't let their needs be known tend to end up being 'martyrs' or 'doormats'. They do whatever work needs to be done, they never say no, they take incredible burdens upon themselves. They often feel resentful about being taken advantage of, and angry with themselves for being a 'doormat'. This anger and resentment and the low opinion they have of themselves can easily turn into depression. And all of this means extra stress and extra headaches.

> 'Asserting yourself doesn't mean that you always get your own way, but at least you avoid that terrible feeling that you've been railroaded into doing something.'

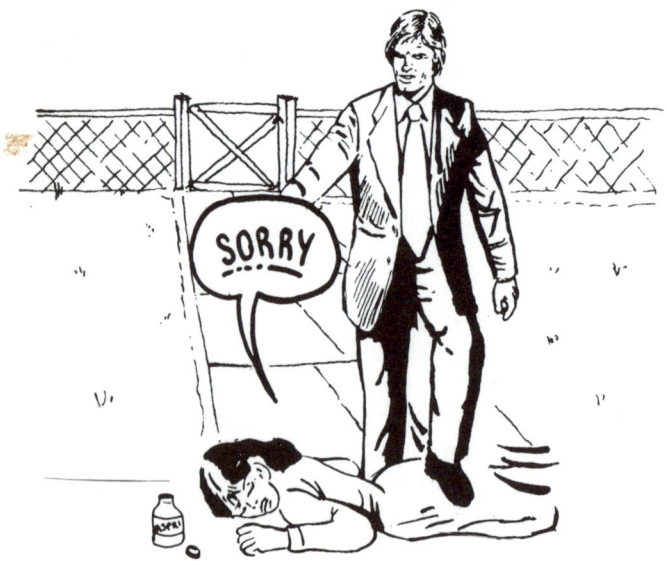

Ask yourself *why* you have difficulty in making your needs known. What are you afraid of? Many people are afraid of being rejected. They think: 'If I say no then they won't want to see me any more'. The truth is that no-one respects a doormat anyway, and they will probably prefer seeing someone who stuck up for themselves. How do you break out of this fear? The best way is to face up to your fear: start asserting yourself, in small ways at first, and see what the reaction is. See if people *do* reject you. Say when you feel you have too much work to do. Say when you need some time off. Say when you are unable to meet a deadline. Even if you don't get what you need, at least you will feel better about yourself.

Things really are that simple, but often people need help in overcoming fears. Find out if there is an *assertiveness group* running near you: some local authorities run them for women. The Redwood Women's Training Association also organises courses throughout Britain: their address is given in the back of this book. Becoming assertive won't turn you into an aggressive selfish person. It might mean that you stop creating extra stress for yourself and that you feel better about yourself and more in control of your life. All of which mean that you cope much better and work more efficiently and have fewer headaches. Indeed, there has been a study that showed that assertiveness training can reduce headaches. If there is not a group near you, I have recommended some reading on how to be more assertive at the end of this book.

Emotional difficulties and headaches

We all get periods of feeling low or feeling worried. Sometimes it seems that the least thing upsets us. This is much more likely if we are tense and finding it difficult to cope. That is why learning relaxation techniques can seem to make you a more 'balanced' person.

'... It has taught me not to let myself get screwed up over unimportant things so in a way has altered my view on life and my own situation.'

Any kind of emotional stress can worsen headaches. So ensuring that your feelings do not run away with you can reduce your headaches, and learning how to relax can help with this. But what about serious emotional problems?

Clinical depression

People who suffer from *clinical depression* very often have headaches. Clinical depression means not only feeling very low but also experiencing a number of changes in your nervous system that alter your pattern of sleep, your appetite, and lower your energy levels and your sex drive. Some experts believe that the depression causes the headaches, and that you can only ease the headaches if you lift the depression. This is certainly a possibility, and indeed some of the chemical changes underlying headaches have also been found in depression. Another possibility is that the sheer emotional tension that depressed people put themselves under causes the headaches. On the other hand, people have also been known to become depressed because of the severity of their headaches, which sometimes limit their lives to an unbearable extent. You can see that it is unwise to jump to any one conclusion.

If you do have problems with depression as well as headaches then it is best to have help for both. Otherwise, it is likely that your headaches will make your depression worse, and vice versa. When you are depressed you are much more likely to think negatively about events, fear the worst, and criticise yourself for your failings – all of which create more stress and make your headaches worse. When your depression has lifted enough for you to feel that you can start to take control of your life once more, then that is the time to start the self-help treatments for headache given in this book. Your doctor or psychiatrist will prescribe antidepressants which may give you the boost that you need. Alternatively, they may refer you to a clinical psychologist if you want an approach that does not rely on drugs.

Anxiety problems

People who have *anxiety problems* also suffer headaches. In this case, it is likely that the anxiety – which is just excessive nervous tension – is causing or worsening the headache. It therefore makes sense to treat the anxiety first. Fortunately, however, many of the non-drug treatments for anxiety problems are similar to the relaxation methods that are discussed in this book. As we have seen in Chapter 3, many of the drugs prescribed for tension headache are tranquillisers used for the treatment of anxiety problems. So if you are receiving help for your anxiety, then it is likely that the same treatments will reduce your headaches. If not, then it certainly wouldn't hurt for you to try the relaxation programme put forward in this book.

Sleep problems and headaches

Sleep is connected with many headaches. Cluster headaches very often occur about 90 minutes after falling asleep, and so may be linked to a certain phase of sleep. Too little sleep can trigger migraines. So can oversleeping, although this may be because you have not eaten for a long while. As discussed in the next chapter, if you go without something you are allergic to for a while then you will suffer 'withdrawal' headaches. As you know from the previous chapter, the same thing happens with caffeine. So it may not be the oversleeping itself, but the doing without your early morning coffee that sets off the headache! Tiredness is, however, a definite trigger for both tension and migraine headaches and this naturally is worsened by poor sleep. When you are tired you find it so much harder to cope with life – so inevitably your stress levels rise. Most headache sufferers have to ensure that they sleep well.

As you may have gathered from the previous chapter, learning relaxation techniques can help with your sleeping; when you are less tense you sleep more deeply. All of us have had nights tossing and turning when we are uptight about something. Regular practice with the relaxation exercises can really help. You can also use the exercises (or parts of them) to get off to sleep at night. If, despite this, you still have problems with getting off to sleep or with waking up during the night, here are a few hints to help you:

- Never lie awake for long periods in your bed.
- Try doing your best to stay awake: this gets rid of the
- worry about not getting any sleep and can make you nod off!
- If you can't sleep get up and make yourself a drink (no caffeine!) and read until you are drowsy.
- Never watch television or read in bed.
- Don't do anything energetic or stimulating for at least an hour before you go to bed.
- Cut out caffeine completely!
- Get more exercise during the day.

Exercise and headaches

Strenuous exercise, such as playing squash or football, can trigger a headache. Often people find that if they take painkillers before their exercise this helps to prevent one. In more serious cases a drug called *indomethacin* is said to help, but your doctor will have to prescribe this. Some experts believe it is not the exertion itself that sets off these headaches but low blood sugar, or *hypoglycaemia*. This can be avoided through dietary changes; it will be discussed more in the next chapter. Other people find that exercise which involves certain movements – for instance, stooping while gardening – sets off a headache. In these cases it is likely that strains on inflexible joints and muscles are the cause. Learning to relax the muscles will help, as will gentle exercises designed to improve suppleness, such as yoga.

In general, fairly mild and non-competitive exercise helps to reduce headaches. If you wear proper shoes to avoid jarring of your bones, brisk walking or jogging is ideal. It probably works because it gives the body a chance to 'burn off' chemicals that have built up as part of the stress reaction. If this isn't done, adrenalin will hang around in the body for a good while, keeping your autonomic arousal high. This makes you feel on edge, and your work and relationships suffer – which leads to more stress. People often find that exercise reduces their emotional tension and makes them sleep better. An added bonus is that a fit person is in general more able to cope with life so is less prone to stress reaction.

Your attitude to your headaches

Pain is a major source of stress. So it follows that your headaches are as well. How can you reduce the stress that comes from pain? There are a number of ways but perhaps the best is our old friend relaxation. When people are anxious they feel more pain; when they are relaxed it just doesn't bother them as much. Pain has two sides – the sensation and how bad it is. People with chronic pain who are on morphine can say where the pain is, whether it is throbbing or steady, and how intense it is: but it doesn't bother them. Relaxation can do the same for headache pain. And when you don't tense against the pain, you don't get into the pain→tension→more pain vicious circle that was discussed in Chapter 2. So the headaches are less intense and shorter. When you next get a headache –

migraine or tension – try not to fight it, but relax and go with it. It will run its course in its own time. These are the reasons why it was suggested in Chapter 4 that you can measure both aspects of pain for your headache diary. Relaxation can help in a similar way to morphine, although it is obviously not as effective. Being less bothered by your headache pain is one measure of improvement. In the long run it will show as fewer headaches because you are not letting yourself be stressed by them.

One recent study has shown that after years of suffering headaches people tend to opt out of life more and more: they are more likely to take to their beds or to stop work during their headaches. This may be because they have learned that this is the best way of helping their pain. These sufferers also tend to start avoiding meeting people, travelling, and other situations that they find stressful. Although this can reduce tension which means fewer headaches, in the long run it counts against the person. It seems that the more people opt out, the more sensitive they get to situations. One study showed that

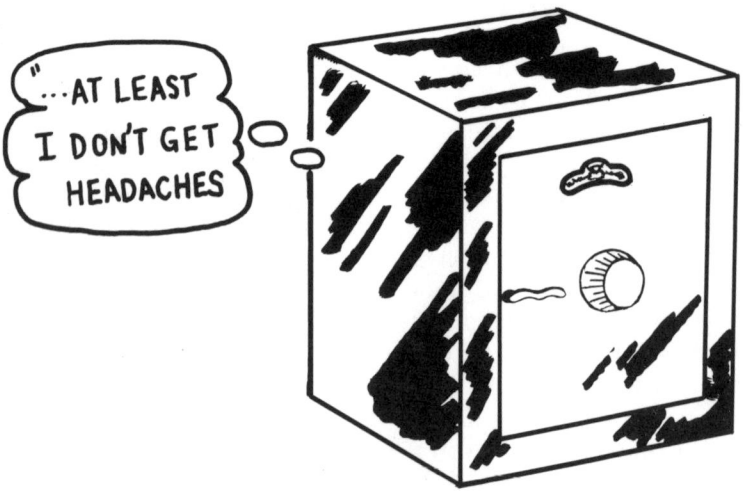

migraine sufferers are more sensitive to noise, even when they don't have a headache. It also makes sense that the more someone avoids social situations and travelling, the more nervous they become about them, and the more difficult it is for them to cope. So you either end up under greater stress, or avoiding more situations. Also, people whose lives are restricted are prone to depression, which can cause headaches.

What does this mean for people with a long-standing headache problem? It means that you should not let your headaches restrict your life. Often, you have no option but to go to bed or to stop work when you have a bad headache. However, avoiding situations that may set off headaches is in the long run counter-productive, as well as spoiling your life. If you already find yourself doing this, it may not be an easy task to get more involved in life once again. The trick is to do it gradually. Get a friend or spouse involved, and draw up a timetable of reintroduction to life. Learning relaxation techniques will help you to face the world again. If things have got bad and you can't manage it on your own, then ask your doctor for specialist help. Clinical psychologists can help with this kind of problem. In most cases, however, you will be able to manage on your own or with help from a close companion. It will be worth it in the long run.

7. Diet, Allergies and Headaches

Most of the research on diet and headaches has concentrated on migraine headaches. The fact that diet is linked to migraine is now well established. However, clinicians who work in this area are also reporting that tension-type headaches can be helped by a change of diet. Nevertheless, it is not known how many tension headache sufferers are helped, or to what degree. Perhaps it is best to say that if you suffer a kind of migraine or if you get migraine-type symptoms then you would be well advised to follow at least some of the suggestions in this chapter. If you get tension headaches then this approach may well be worth pursuing if you do not achieve the improvements that you were hoping for from the relaxation techniques.

Food and Headaches

Many people are aware that if they eat certain foods then they will get a headache. Cheese, chocolate, oranges and red wine are commonly reported triggers of migraine attacks. However, few people will get full relief from simply cutting out these foods. Some *do*, so try it; you will have an idea of which are the most important to avoid from your headache diary. Other common triggers are discussed later in this chapter, and include smoking, the contraceptive pill, caffeine and alcohol. Many people find that their headaches are helped considerably by cutting out all of these triggers. Try it and see.

The main part of this chapter, however, will discuss a more radical dietary approach than simply cutting out triggers. This involves the idea of food *allergies*. You can attempt part or all of this approach on your own. You may, however, find that you need assistance, in which case contact one of the organisations given in the appendix for the address of your nearest practitioner. Your best option is to seek out a specialist; these are called *clinical ecologists*. The ideas and methods discussed in this chapter are not yet widely known or used, so it is unlikely that your doctor will be familiar with them.

Some medical allergists will not recognise or agree with the concept of food allergies as discussed in this chapter. This is because the types of bodily changes that have been identified in 'established' allergies have yet to be shown in the kind of food allergies that are discussed here. It is for this reason that some specialists prefer the term *food sensitivities*. To avoid confusion with many of the popular books written in this field, however, I will continue to use the term *allergy*. This does not imply any specific bodily change.

The remainder of this chapter concerns *hypoglycaemia*, or low blood sugar, considered by some a possible cause of headaches. This again is somewhat controversial, some doctors claiming that it doesn't even exist. Nevertheless, the hypoglycaemia approach has helped many headache sufferers.

A word of warning: with all these approaches it is vital to make sure that your long-term diet is balanced and adequate in terms of minerals, vitamins, carbohydrates, fibre, and so on. Your doctor will be able to advise on this.

Allergies

You might assume that allergies are easily recognised. If you start sneezing when cats are around, you are allergic to cats or something on them. If you get a migraine whenever you eat cheese, you are allergic to cheese. But many allergies are *masked* and are not that simple. If you regularly consume something that you are allergic to (an *allergen*), your body adapts to it, but only to a certain extent. The continual aggravation by the allergen can cause many nagging symptoms such as continual tiredness, aches, high blood pressure, and frequent tension-type headaches. However, as your body becomes used to the allergen, you develop symptoms if you do without it; these can be called 'withdrawal' effects. This is when more serious headaches can occur, particularly migraines. Many other 'withdrawal' symptoms are possible apart from headaches, and may include aches and pains, fatigue and depression. By consuming the allergen the body can stave these off.

You may see the parallel with drug and alcohol addiction here. In many senses the body does become addicted to the allergen; you will find yourself wanting the allergen a great deal of the time. Foods or drinks that people crave or eat a lot of are good candidates for allergens. If, however, the body is not in regular contact with an allergen, and so does not become adapted to it, then when the substance is eaten a dramatic reaction is often seen. This may be the case when people identify triggers for their migraines, such as cheese or chocolate.

When you regularly eat or breathe something that you are allergic to, you may never realise your allergy but suffer many nagging, constant symptoms including headaches. Because it is when you do *without* the allergen that you get a really bad headache, you will probably never realise the connection.

Allergies can also change over a person's lifetime. You may have heard of people growing out of hay fever or asthma, or developing them later on in life. A substance that caused no problems when you first came into contact with it, may after many years develop into an allergen. Some people can think back . . . 'Yes, my headaches started when I first started smoking', but most can't. This is especially true since most allergens are very common foods that people eat from their first year of life.

Common allergies

The most common foods that people seem to be allergic to are not well-known triggers such as cheese or chocolate. The worst culprits are said to be some of the most commonly eaten foods: wheat, corn, dairy products, eggs, yeast and sugar. Many clinical ecologists believe that these foods are a problem because they are recent introductions to mankind's diet. Our digestive systems may not yet be geared up to dealing with them in any quantity. When you consider how prevalent these foods are in our everyday diet, it is not surprising that they cause our bodies problems. For instance, corn in some form is in most processed foods. Look for the term 'edible starch' – that is probably corn. Cornflour is in most mass-produced cakes, biscuits, custard, canned soups, much Chinese food, and so on. It is used as a binder in most tablets. Corn oil is very often used for frying and as an ingredient in margarine, where it is often called 'vegetable oil'. Glucose can be made from corn and is an ingredient in most soft drinks and chocolates and sweets or candies. So you can see that corn is an ingredient in a major part of our modern diet.

Other common allergens are not foods but are substances that are breathed in. Of particular relevance to headaches are *petrochemicals*. These are gases such as natural gas, coal gas, fumes from petrol or gasoline, and less obvious ones such as those from perfumes or nail varnish. Some people notice how they develop headaches during a long car journey, and attribute this to the stress of driving. This may be so, but an allergy to petrol or diesel fumes can be responsible – a history of car sickness, but no sea sickness, would suggest this. However, in general, allergies to foods are more important in causing headaches than allergies to gases. In one important study 93% of children who suffered from migraines became symptom-free on a corrected diet. Unfortunately, a similarly careful study has yet to be done with adults, but this may be a matter of time.

Finding out whether allergies cause your headaches

The simplest and most reliable way of finding out whether allergies are causing your headaches is to go on an *elimination diet*. This involves eating only foods that are unlikely to be allergens for six or seven days. If allergies are relevant for you, then you should not only be headache-free but also be rid of those less severe, nagging symptoms such as aching limbs, tiredness, low spirits, and so on. The idea is then to gradually reintroduce foods and see which foods you are allergic to. The elimination diet is tackled in more detail in the next section.

There are many other methods available to diagnose food allergies. Most of these, unfortunately, are unreliable and untested. There are two types of tests on blood samples. One is called the *radio-allergo sorbent test*, or RAST test, and the other *cytotoxic testing*. Basically, the RAST test looks at the number of antibodies that react to the food being tested, and the cytotoxic test looks at the effects of foods on certain blood cells. Both depend on the judgement of the clinician doing the test and can therefore be inaccurate. The RAST in particular can be expensive. Other less scientific methods involve using hair samples and seeing which way they rotate when weighted (*radionics*) and measuring muscle strength before and after eating the suspected food.

Perhaps the most commonly used test is *skin prick testing* or the *scratch test*. In this, small samples of suspected allergens are pricked into your skin, which is supposed to react if you are allergic to the substance. Unfortunately, recent evidence shows that this method is not satisfactory for food allergies, although it can be useful for identifying inhaled allergies.

There are two satisfactory alternatives to the elimination diet. Both involve taking varying doses of the suspected allergens and watching out for symptoms. The first involves putting drops of the food under the tongue, where it is quickly absorbed; this is called *sublingual provocative testing*. Unfortunately, many foods are absorbed only slowly, especially cereals such as corn or wheat. A good description of the use of this technique is given in the classic book *Not All in the Mind* by Richard Mackarness. The second type of test involves injections of suspect substances into the skin, *intradermal provocative testing*. An advantage of this procedure is that the skin reaction can be used to demonstrate allergic reactions in addition to the production of any symptoms. This method also produces an accurate dose of the allergen that can be used for neutralising a person's allergy – this will be discussed later in this chapter.

An elimination diet

The withdrawal phase

An elimination diet has two stages. In the first, or *withdrawal phase*, you eat only foods that are low allergy risks. This lasts for one week. Obviously the fewer kinds of food you eat, the lower the chance that you will be eating something you are allergic to. In the second phase, the *reintroduction period*, you gradually start eating other foods to see if they set off an allergic reaction. For the withdrawal phase, the foods that seem to have the lowest risk for allergies are:

- pears
- lamb
- carrots
- courgettes
- runner and french beans.

The following foods are also fairly safe, and can be included if you feel that you cannot put up with eating only the above foods for a week. *Never* include anything that you normally eat more often than every four days, even if it is on the list – this may be an allergen. The fairly safe foods are:

- white fish

- swedes, turnips and parsnips

- avocado pears

- cabbage and broccoli but *only* if organically grown.

It is best to eat only organically-grown fruit and vegetables in general, because some people are allergic to the chemical sprays that are used. Drink *only* bottled water during this withdrawal phase.

For one week, eat only these low-risk foods. You can eat as much of them as you want. Use *no* butter, margarine, oils, pepper, spices, and so on, to cook with. Pure sea salt is allowed. You may find that you become quite inventive at thinking up dishes or ways of cooking the foods. The fat that runs off the lamb can be used for sautéeing the courgettes, for instance.

It is also advisable during the elimination diet to stop all the medications that you can, but ask your doctor for advice about this. All tablets contain binders, fillers or flavourings that you may be allergic to. It is particularly important that you discontinue taking contraceptive pills and ergotamine. You must also *stop smoking*. It would be sensible to stop these three or four weeks before the elimination diet. You will then know how much these drugs have been affecting your headaches in comparison with any allergies. Beware of the rebound headaches you can get when you stop taking ergotamine (see Chapter 3).

If the withdrawal phase has had no effect by the sixth day, allergies are not a problem for you. For people who do have food or chemical allergies, however, there will be *withdrawal* effects. These effects are different in different people. They will involve the symptoms that the allergy has been causing all this while: a very bad headache or extreme tiredness, for instance. Aches and depression are also common. This withdrawal headache generally comes by the evening of the first or the morning of the second day and lasts into the fifth or sixth day. The headache is often so bad it will be tempting to take painkillers or ergotamine; try to resist this. It will be followed by a feeling of wellbeing that you probably have never experienced before – you just *know* that you won't get a headache. This pattern is a fairly sure sign that allergies are part of your problem.

Reintroducing foods

After this withdrawal phase, you then need to reintroduce foods one by one. If a particular food does not produce symptoms, it is passed as 'safe' and can be eaten from then on. You can reintroduce a different food at every meal, providing there has been a gap of five or six hours so that symptoms can develop if the food is an allergen (cereals are a special case, however, as you will see).

By the end of the withdrawal phase you will probably crave alternative foods. You may also, however, be enjoying the feeling of wellbeing. For the first few days, then, it may be worthwhile introducing other low-risk foods. These include melon, apples, grapes, lettuce, rice and chicken. They can also include any food that you don't regularly eat, because this is unlikely to have been a cause of your headaches. Once all these are reintroduced, your diet can become quite varied!

When you reintroduce a food that you are allergic to, you will have a reaction more extreme than normal because your body is no longer adapted to the allergen, having gone without it for a week. You may have a very severe headache, for instance. This will generally happen within two or three hours of eating the food. Some foods, however, are absorbed much more slowly by the body. This is true of cereals such as wheat or corn. When reintroducing cereals, allow a couple of days for the symptoms to develop. So for these two days, eat only 'allowed' foods plus the cereal. If there is no reaction in two days, then that particular cereal can be passed as safe. Remember to eat only *pure* cereal, however, unless the other ingredients have already been passed as safe. In this respect, it may be wise to test your reaction to sugars fairly early, since cereals in the form of breakfast cereals generally contain sugars. Remember that cane sugar and beet sugar should be tested separately.

Whatever you do, *don't* introduce foods like bread or cake to the diet. Mixtures such as these are strictly forbidden. If you find that you react badly to bread, for instance, does that mean that you are allergic to the wheat? the yeast? the sugar? preservatives? Or what? So you can see that only *single* foods are of use in identifying allergies.

If you do find an allergen:

Don't stop the diet there! Most people are sensitive to more than one food.

Don't 'test' a similar food within five days. For instance, if you react to lemons don't test oranges within five days; if milk causes a problem, avoid all dairy products for five days. This is because one food from within a 'family' may mask the reaction to another, in the same way as eating an allergen regularly masks or staves off a dramatic allergic reaction.

Make sure you are symptom-free before testing another food.

If you seem to have a mild reaction, or if the symptoms do not include a headache but are less obvious (for instance depressed feelings or lethargy), then you may like to re-test the food later on. You can do this, but make sure you do not eat it again for at least five days, to avoid possible masking effects.

Diet, Allergies and Headaches

A few hints to help you with your diet:

- Make sure you choose the right time for the elimination diet. Although the 'withdrawal' phase lasts only a week, if food allergies are relevant for you, your diet will be quite restricted for many weeks after. So avoid a time when you have to go to dinner parties, weddings, and so on.
- Make up the menu in advance for each week. Search through recipe books and adapt recipes. Try to make it as interesting as possible.
- Avoid buying tempting foods. Make a shopping list in advance, and don't shop when you're feeling hungry! If you have a family, involve them in what you are doing. They don't have to eat what you do but they can provide emotional support.
- If you have a partner, involve him or her in the diet. They may have less severe symptoms such as a low mood or tiredness that may be the result of allergies.
- If you find you cannot stick to your diet, don't get too upset. Many people cannot manage to give up smoking, for instance, even for a few weeks. The elimination diet will still be of value in identifying food allergies. If you find that you cannot resist eating cakes or other mixtures during the withdrawal phase, start again and make sure that you can't get to them! If you eat these kinds of foods in the reintroduction phase and you don't get any reaction, then you know that the ingredients are safe (remember to allow two days for the flour). If you do get a reaction, then after a five-day gap you will have to test *all* of the ingredients separately.
- If all else fails, you can seek out a doctor interested in clinical ecology who can try intradermal provocative testing.

Dealing with your allergies

The most direct method of dealing with allergies is to avoid the allergen. This is easy with less common foods. Unfortunately the most common allergens are cereals, sugar and dairy products all of which are very hard to avoid. Nevertheless, many sufferers manage to avoid their forbidden foods quite successfully, having decided that their headaches provide a big enough incentive.

A relatively new alternative is called *neutralisation* or *desensitisation*. Curiously, when you give a certain dose of an allergen to the sufferer, it appears to neutralise the allergy. Somehow, the person is 'inoculated' against the allergen for a while. If this dose is applied in drops under the tongue, the person is protected for perhaps five or six hours; if it is injected beneath the skin, this protection lasts for up to two days. When a person is allergic to more than one substance then all the allergens can be put into each dose. Furthermore, it is said that about two years of this neutralising therapy results in a permanent resistance to the allergen. This method is enthusiastically recommended by some clinical ecologists, and of course offers many advantages over simply avoiding the allergens. The scientific evidence that is available seems to support the effectiveness of this method, but a note of caution should be sounded since the amount of this evidence is small.

There are a number of clinics that offer neutralisation and desensitisation therapy in Great Britain and many in the USA. Their addresses can be found from one of the national organisations of clinical ecology which are listed in the back of this book.

Intestinal thrush

Some clinical ecologists believe that intestinal thrush is central to many allergy problems. For a full discussion of this, John Mansfield's book *The Migraine Revolution* is valuable reading. Thrush is a type of fungus that lives in everyone's intestines or gut. It is the same fungus that often infects babies' mouths or women's vaginas, causing irritation and a white discharge. Problems are said to occur when the numbers of a certain form of thrush greatly increase in the intestine. They produce a kind of poison that can worsen allergies. Thrush also makes the gut walls more 'leaky' so that improperly digested foods can get into the blood stream, making allergies more likely.

Luckily, intestinal thrush can be easily and safely treated using a drug called *Nystatin*. Some people have found remarkable improvements in their symptoms following this treatment. Unfortunately, there are no quick clinical tests that can diagnose intestinal thrush problems. You should know, however, that the following can make you vulnerable to thrush: prolonged or repeated courses of antibiotics and long-standing use of cortisone, cortisone-type drugs (steroids) or a contraceptive pill containing oestrogen. Signs of an infection are said to be: indigestion-type symptoms, constipation, irritation of the anal passage, bloated abdomen, recurrent vaginal thrush, cystitis and fungal-type rashes over the body. Your doctor may be able to help if you suspect a thrush infection. Treating this, in itself, may be enough to reduce your headaches.

Other Factors That May Cause Headaches

Alcohol

Many people's headaches are triggered by alcoholic drinks. It could be that the alcohol itself is setting off a reaction. However, if only certain drinks trigger a headache then it is possible that you are allergic to one of the ingredients. Because the allergen is in a solution of alcohol, it is very rapidly absorbed into the body and has an almost immediate effect: these have been called, rightly, 'turbo-charged' allergens.

Smoking

Cigarette smoke can cause or contribute to headaches. One study showed that 13% of non-smoking migraine sufferers who avoided cheese, chocolate, citrus fruits, alcohol and other people's cigarette smoke became headache-free. However, 53% of a similar group of migraine sufferers who were smokers became headache-free when asked to give up smoking as well as these other triggers. Smoking was obviously causing migraines in many of these people. This may be surprising because most people's headaches do not coincide with the start of their smoking habit. A sensitivity to cigarettes appears to develop over a person's lifetime. This may or may not be an allergy, but that doesn't really matter if giving up smoking cures your headaches. If you do smoke, you would be well advised to try stopping, at least temporarily.

'The Pill'

A few women develop headaches when they first start taking a contraceptive pill and, in general, they change the kind of pill until one is found that does not have such side-effects. The progesterone-only pill which contains no oestrogen seems to be less prone to cause headaches than the ordinary 'combined' pill. Some women *develop* a reaction to the pill, sometimes many years after starting to take it. In the same study as the one on smoking, 33% of women who gave up the pill as well as the other triggers became headache-free, as opposed to the 13% who were not on the pill. Unfortunately, sometimes the headaches persist for months after the pill is stopped, and about one in ten women continue to suffer headaches indefinitely. Again, trial-and-error is the best tactic here: change your method of contraception and, using your headache diary, see if there is any reduction in your headaches.

Food 'triggers'

As you already know, migraines are often set off by eating cheese, chocolate or oranges, and by drinking red wine. Some experts believe that a substance called *tyramine* that is in each of these foods causes headaches. Other foods that contain a lot of tyramine are: yoghurt, bananas and well-hung or 'jugged' meat. If you find that cheese, chocolate, citrus fruits and red wine all cause migraines, you may be reacting to tyramine and it would be worth trying to cut out all tyramine-rich foods. If you react to only one or two, however, an allergy to the particular food is more likely.

Other substances that can trigger headaches and which are found in many foods are *additives*. Common culprits are *nitrites* and *nitrates*: these are chemicals that can swell your blood vessels and so cause vascular headaches. They are often added to hot dogs, canned meat, bacon and cured meats like salami to make them look red and 'appetising'. If you buy these kinds of foods, have a look at the ingredients on the packet and see if nitrites or nitrates have been added. Then chart them as a possible trigger in your headache diary. Do the same also with *monosodium glutamate*, which can also set off headaches in many people. This is a 'flavour enhancer' that is found in many processed foods and in Chinese food – try charting Chinese food as a possible trigger.

Hypoglycaemia

Some people's headaches are due to low blood sugar, or *hypoglycaemia*. This condition has been said to underlie many different physical and psychological problems. Indeed, hypoglycaemia can produce a great variety of symptoms and mimic other health problems. It can also uncover sensitivities or allergies to foods, so that if your hypoglycaemia were dealt with the allergy would also go.

How do you know that you have blood sugar problems? Unfortunately it is difficult to tell, because the hypoglycaemia can produce so many different symptoms. However, the following signs may be clues:

- if your headaches begin a few hours after eating, or when you don't eat;
- extreme tiredness;
- depressed moods and irritability;
- overactivity and poor concentration;
- feeling faint;
- shaking;
- cold sweats and panic;
- allergies;
- stomach or digestive problems;

and particularly:

- if any of the above symptoms get worse if you miss a meal and get better with cigarettes, alcohol, caffeine, and especially sweet foods;
- if you have a craving for sweet foods, foods high in carbohydrates, and stimulants.

Some doctors use a special test called a *glucose tolerance test* to see whether a person has low blood sugar problems. In this test you are given glucose on an empty stomach and a series of blood tests to chart how the body deals with it. This test may not be 100% accurate, however.

It may appear odd that people can develop low blood sugar on a Western diet which is so high in sugar and carbohydrates (a ready source of blood sugar). What seems to happen is that a number of factors unbalance the body's system for keeping blood sugar levels constant. These factors include eating lots of sugar and refined carbohydrates, taking many stimulants, and being under too much stress.

Stimulants and stress both cause the adrenal glands to produce *adrenalin*. The adrenal glands also make available sugars that have been stored by the body for 'emergencies' – this is the fuel that gives you extra energy when you are anxious. At the same time as the adrenal gland is doing this, the body produces *insulin* to keep the level of sugar in the blood down to normal levels. However, if the adrenal gland is not operating properly – if it has been exhausted by too much stress and too many stimulants, for instance – then it will not be able to call forth the body's stored sugars very efficiently. So you develop a craving for sugar and carbohydrates. At the same time your body has still produced the insulin, so lowering your blood sugar levels. Eating carbohydrates helps in the short term by boosting your blood sugar levels but in the long term stimulates the production of more insulin, lowering your blood sugar levels further. So you crave more carbohydrates, and so on, leading to hypoglycaemia.

Many doctors and experts do not believe in the existence of hypoglycaemia. They believe that the body's system of keeping blood sugar levels constant is so good that only disease and certain drugs can upset it. Because of the difficulties in diagnosing hypoglycaemia, there are few scientific studies as yet. However, the number of different people whose symptoms fit into the hypoglycaemic pattern and who are helped by changing their diet suggests that this may be a common problem. If you feel that low blood sugar may be a problem for you, discuss the possibility with your doctor. It may be possible to have a glucose tolerance test. If not, see if the recommended dietary changes given below make an improvement in your headaches – you should see benefits within a month. If it does help, continue for at least three months and preferably indefinitely. And even if it doesn't help your headaches, you will be more healthy for it!

How to help hypoglycaemia

- Cut out all stimulants: this means caffeine and smoking.
- Avoid alcoholic drinks.
- Learn relaxation exercises (see Chapter 5).
- Take regular gentle exercise (see Chapter 6).

Change your diet:

- eat little and often; five or six small meals a day, and a snack before bedtime
- avoid white sugar, white flour, and white rice: so cakes, sweets or candy, and white bread are definitely out!
- reduce the amount of sweet and fatty foods in your diet
- eat more fresh vegetables and fibre-rich food, and fresh fruits (but avoid sweet fruit juices).

Many of these recommendations are similar to those in previous chapters. When you are learning relaxation exercises you must cut out stimulants. Many of the foods that you must avoid to improve hypoglycaemia are also allergens. Alcoholic drinks are common triggers of migraine, as is hunger. Gentle exercise, also, is recommended in the previous chapter. So it would seem sensible to follow this regime, regardless of your headache type.

8. Alternatives

Alternative Approaches

In this last chapter I will discuss various different approaches that you may want to try if the methods in this book do not appeal or work for you. Many of them come under the umbrella of 'alternative medicines', which are lumped together only because they are not generally part of our present health system. All of these approaches are similar in one respect, however. They treat the *whole* person. In other words, they don't consider the mind as being separate from the body; they believe that a person has the potential to heal him- or herself, and is not merely a 'patient' to be healed by a doctor. Because alternative approaches view the mind as being important to 'physical' problems, there is much more emphasis on talking to you and achieving some kind of relationship. The practitioner of alternative medicine will spend a lot of time with you. Each person is viewed as an individual case, and so medical diagnoses will not be seen as very relevant.

Although in past years such therapies have been scorned by many doctors, in recent times many medical practitioners are accepting and even training in alternative approaches. The issue of training is particularly important when considering alternative medicine. Although most approaches have an organisation that oversees many of its practitioners, there will always be unscrupulous people with unsuitable training who practise. If you are considering using one of these approaches – and many come highly recommended by people who have been helped enormously – then make sure you see a properly trained person. Your best bet is to contact one of the national organisations listed in the back of this book. It is not necessary to seek out a medical doctor who has trained in an alternative approach, but it is always wise to inform your doctor if you are going to try alternative medicine. The approach may not be compatible with medical treatment that you are having.

The one great advantage of 'alternative' medicine is that you risk very little, apart from your money. With properly trained practitioners, there are no dangers or side-effects, unlike conventional medicine. This is because of the emphasis on the person healing themselves, and not being 'cured' by drugs or operations.

Acupuncture

Acupuncture is a form of treatment that involves sticking needles into the skin. Perhaps the idea of this frightens or repels you. However, it is rarely painful and indeed many people find the sensation pleasurable in some way. The needles generally don't even draw blood because they are so thin. When properly sterilised, the needles cannot transmit infection and do no harm.

Acupuncture is based on an ancient system of medicine developed in China that is totally different from Western medicine. In traditional Chinese medicine, acupuncture (and the massage that is its equivalent, *acupressure*) is just one of many different therapies that are based on the same system. Others are various forms of massage, herbal medicine, dietary changes, manipulating the body, and exercises. The Chinese believe that illness is caused by the interruption of the natural flow of energy along certain paths. The acupuncture needles and acupressure massage are said to restore the flow along these energy pathways.

The acupuncturist has a complicated system of diagnosis that bears little resemblance to our own. He or she uses various methods for diagnosing, including a detailed history of the problem and an examination. The examination pays particular attention to your pulse – there are said to be six different pulses in each wrist. Each pulse tells something to the practitioner about the flow of energy in your body. Also, the tongue may be examined, and your head. All this probably does not make sense to you, but it would be unwise to reject it simply because it does not match the Western system of medicine. What matters most is if it works.

Treatment involves seeing the acupuncturist perhaps once a week for a few months; however, if you feel no benefit after three or four sessions then leave it there. At each meeting a few needles will be inserted in the important places – most often in the lower arms and legs – and left in for 10 or 20 minutes. Some acupuncturists use the ears for putting their needles in; the idea is that there is a 'map' of the body's energy pathways on the ear. Perhaps surprisingly, many claim this method to be just as effective as the traditional approach.

There is also a Western equivalent of traditional Chinese acupuncture. This approach aims more to relieve symptoms rather than cure the causes. It attempts to lock into the body's own system of pain control (which traditional acupuncture might do anyway), sometimes using a weak electric current down the needle. Some doctors and physiotherapists have been trained in this *medical acupuncture*.

Does acupuncture work? Well, there is more and more scientific evidence to show that it does work, and with many different problems. Most of the research has studied medical acupuncture, but there are numerous case histories to show the effectiveness of the traditional approach – which is just as well, because this is the approach that you are likely to come across if you decide to give it a go. Acupuncture seems to be effective for both preventing and treating headaches. Unfortunately, yet again, it is not known how to identify those that can be helped. You just have to try it and see. But make sure that you see a practitioner who has adequate training: the national organisations listed in the back of this book will point you in the right direction.

Osteopathy and chiropractic

Both these kinds of treatment involve the therapist moving and adjusting your bone structure. Both concentrate on your spine, although an osteopath also manipulates other bones in your body. Chiropractic pays particular attention to trapped nerves. Many headaches seem to be caused by problems in the neck and spine, and these two methods attempt to deal with these causes. Although osteopathy and chiropractic differ in their background and approach, to the lay person they are quite similar. There have been many instances of people's headaches being reduced or cured altogether using these techniques, although few scientific studies have been done. They may work best in cases where the person also has neck pain or back trouble, as well as headaches; also if the headaches started after some injury, or if poor posture is involved.

The Alexander technique

This technique teaches you to improve your posture through a number of special exercises. It is said to help many different problems and to make you more relaxed. It can relax you because your body holds itself under tension to maintain a poor posture, whereas good posture is naturally relaxing. Alexander technique may help headaches both through relieving the muscle tension and through correcting imbalances in the bone structure. There have been a few reports of it reducing headaches, but no scientific studies as yet.

Homeopathy

Homeopathic medicine is another system of medicine that bears little resemblance to ordinary medicine. It has ancient roots but has re-emerged in the last 150 years. It is based on the principle of 'like treats like', rather similar to vaccination. If we want to protect ourselves from some disease we inject a mild form of the disease into our body so that it learns to protect itself. Homeopathy also uses our body's own ability to heal itself, but in a different way. It does this by introducing to the body a substance that, if taken in quantity, produces similar symptoms to whatever needs to be cured. So if you are treating headaches, the homeopath might use a substance that causes headaches when eaten in greater amounts. Very small quantities are used as remedies.

Homeopaths do not just treat the obvious symptoms but also the underlying causes, so the remedy may not be that simple: the substance chosen has to duplicate a whole symptom 'picture'. There seem to be various types of people and headaches that fit into particular 'pictures'. There are therefore some remedies that are commonly given for headaches, and which are available in health food shops. There is no risk involved in taking these because the doses are so small; and no side-effects. However, in general it is better to go to a skilled homeopath who can select a remedy especially for you.

If you do decide to see a homeopath, you will find that at the first interview you will be talking a great deal about yourself. You may take away a remedy, often only one or very few tablets. Some people are disappointed in this, but it may be all that is needed. Your body's reaction to this remedy will give more information to the homeopath, who then be in a position to prescribe a further remedy, and so on until the roots of the problem are dealt with.

Homeopathy is growing in popularity and is becoming more accepted by the medical establishment. There is a good deal of scientific evidence for its effectiveness, and many satisfied customers. In Britain people can sometimes get homeopathic treatment on the National Health Service, and many doctors have further training in homeopathy. Some homeopaths believe, however, that their system of medicine does not sit happily with ordinary medicine: you cannot use a bit of one system and a bit of the other. There are indeed many good lay homeopaths available; addresses of the national organisations are in the back of this book.

Herbal remedies

There is a long history of the treatment of headaches with herbal remedies. One particular herb has attracted much scientific attention recently; this is a member of the chrysanthemum family called *feverfew* – its Latin name is *tanacetum parthenium*. This has been shown in one recent large-scale study to be very effective at preventing migraines. In fact, one third of the sufferers taking it had no further migraines at all; three quarters had some benefit. All that was required was to eat between one and five leaves of feverfew every day. Sore mouths were the only side-effect! Feverfew is now available in tablet form so even this minor side-effect can be avoided. It is highly recommended to anyone suffering from migraine (and is also beneficial in arthritis). However, this should not be the *only* treatment, even if it is totally effective. It does not appear to treat the causes of the headaches but rather stops the symptoms from appearing. If you do not deal with the causes (particularly stress, food sensitivities and hypoglycaemia) then the chances are that other symptoms will appear.

One other herbal remedy should be mentioned. This is *oil of evening primrose* which has been found to ease headaches linked to the menstrual cycle. You should be able to tell whether your headaches worsen with your menstrual cycle from your headache diary. Oil of evening primrose is available from chemists and health food shops in a form called Efamol, which unfortunately is quite expensive. It may, however, help with other period problems such as pains, fluid retention and low mood. An alternative remedy for menstrual headaches is vitamin B6, or Pyridoxine. Some women have found this effective when taken in doses of about 150mg a day. Take this daily, starting from three days before the time your menstrual headaches usually start, and continuing until the time when they usually ease off.

Hypnosis

Hypnosis has a place in our folklore as a rather strange, mystical power, and many people are wary of it. Images of being hypnotised against one's will and being made to do awful or embarrassing things understandably make people nervous. The idea of someone else being in control of you *is* frightening. Fortunately, the kind of hypnosis used in therapy is far removed from stage acts and horror movies. In therapeutic hypnosis, you have to *want* to be hypnotised. You are in control. Anyone can break out of the hypnotic state if they want to. There is no magic about it, and hypnotherapists do not need any special powers or have magnetic personalities. The hypnotic state used in treatment is a form of deep relaxation, similar to how you feel just before going to sleep.

To achieve the hypnotic state you have to use an *induction* procedure, like concentrating on an object or on your breathing. The hypnotherapist will then suggest that you close your eyes and let yourself drift into hypnosis. When you are in this state your psychological barriers are down so that you are open to various *suggestions* from the therapist. These suggestions might help you deal with stress, or the headache pain itself. There is generally a carry-over effect whereby these suggestions work in everyday life. You may also be taught *autohypnosis* so that you can reach a hypnotic state yourself.

There is a great deal of evidence that hypnosis can be helpful with a whole range of psychological and physical problems, including headaches. It is probably worthwhile, however, to give the treatments in this book a good try for a few months before going to a hypnotherapist. In many ways the approach is similar – and cheaper. If you do decide to try hypnosis, do make sure that you go to a registered practitioner. This field is particularly full of poorly-trained and bogus therapists. Some medical doctors and clinical psychologists have done specialist training in hypnosis, and good lay hypnotherapists are also worth seeking out. Contact one of the professional organisations listed in the back of this book for details.

Biofeedback

About 20 years ago it was found that people could learn to control things about their bodies that were once thought totally automatic (this has been known to Eastern civilisations for thousands of years). They could control their heart rate, their muscle tension, their blood vessels, their brain waves... it seemed that there was no limit! All people required was a machine to tell them what they were doing: a machine that could measure heart rate, for instance, and *feed back* to the person how fast his heart was going. So there would be a meter, for instance, or some kind of read-out. Once the person knew what his body was doing then he could control it – to a certain extent. The possibilities were endless, or so it was believed. We could teach tension headache sufferers to lower their head and neck muscle tension! Or migraine sufferers to control their blood systems!

Since that 'honeymoon' period, the limitations of feeding back to the person information about his body, *biofeedback*, have become more obvious. Control over the body can be achieved, but it is not easy. Many people cannot do it to order, and many others cannot translate what they have learned to 'real life' – they cannot do without the machines.

Over the years, three kinds of biofeedback have been used with headache sufferers. Muscle tension feedback, generally from the forehead, has been used with tension headache cases: the idea was to raise people's awareness of, and to reduce, forehead muscle tension. With migraine cases, two different kinds of biofeedback have been tried: learning to warm your hands, and learning to reduce the blood flow in the arteries to your head. When your hands are warm that means that you are relaxed so a migraine is less likely. Learning to reduce the blood flow to your head was thought to be useful because the person could then stop the pain due to swollen blood vessels (we now know that migraine is more complicated, and probably involves the pain 'gate': see Chapter 2).

Biofeedback can indeed help with headaches but it is no more effective than relaxation training. Biofeedback machinery is expensive. However, we do not yet know what kinds of people and headaches are helped by biofeedback; perhaps it can help people that relaxation can't, and vice versa. This is doubtful, however, because it seems that biofeedback has its main effect through relaxing the person anyway. Learning to relax without a machine means that you cannot become dependent on one and you don't have to pay for it. So all in all, it would seem unwise to try biofeedback unless it is freely available, or as a last resort. In Great Britain it can be difficult to track down biofeedback facilities; your best bet would be to contact the local department of clinical psychology. In the USA it appears an easier task; ask your doctor.

Meditation

Meditation has been part of the religious and spiritual life of many Eastern cultures for a very long time. In recent times it has become more popular in the West, often for its 'personal growth' potential. *Transcendental meditation* is one such approach. As far as headache is concerned, its use for relaxation purposes is more interesting. Meditation has been adapted for clinical use in some centres in the States, and indeed many relaxation approaches have similarities to meditation. In most kinds of meditation, the person is required to clear his or her mind and to concentrate on one thing: an object, or a word that is repeated inside the person's head. This can be difficult for someone whose mind keeps racing. That is why relaxation techniques that aim to reduce *physical* tension, like the ones in this book, are often preferable. You can see, however, the similarity to relaxation exercises. Concentrating on your breathing, for instance, is recommended in this book. You are advised to start with the more straightforward relaxation exercises in this book before trying meditation. If the philosophy surrounding a meditation approach appeals to you, go ahead; you may indeed find that it also reduces your headaches.

Community relaxation groups

If you have difficulty in learning relaxation exercises on your own, there may be a relaxation group running near you. Your health authority or education authority may organise such groups, and a charity called Relaxation for Living also runs many. The address for this charity is in the back of this book; contact them for your nearest group. The type of exercise taught will probably be progressive relaxation (see Chapter 5). You may find that emotional support from other group members, and having to report back your progress, mean that you find it easier to practise the exercises.

One last word of advice – whatever approach you try, give it a good go. The benefits will only come given time. If home practice is required, make sure you practise regularly. If one approach does not succeed, try another. You will find relief in the end.

Useful Addresses

If you intend to contact any of these organisations, enclose a stamped addressed envelope with your enquiry. Some organisations may also require modest payment for their services.

ACUPUNCTURE

British Acupuncture Association and Register Limited
34 Alderney Street
London SW1V 4EU
Tel: 01-834 1012

British Medical Acupuncture Society
67-69 Chancery Lane
London WC2 1AF

The College of Traditional Chinese Acupuncture
Tao House
Queensway
Leamington Spa
Warwickshire
CV31 3LZ
Tel: 0926 22121

The first of these organisations holds a general register of approved practitioners; the British Medical Acupuncture Society lists only medically-qualified acupuncturists, who are trained in 'medical' acupuncture. As seen in Chapter 8, this is a somewhat different approach to traditional Chinese acupuncture, aiming more for relief of symptoms rather than a cure. If you are more interested in traditional approaches, contact the British Acupuncture Association or the College of Traditional Chinese Acupuncture.

THE ALEXANDER TECHNIQUE

The Society of Teachers of the Alexander Technique
10 London House
266 Fulham Road
London SW10 9EL

STAT have a list of 350 approved members who have all undergone a three-year training. They do not see the Alexander Technique as an alternative medicine, but rather as working alongside conventional medicine.

ALLERGIES AND CLINICAL ECOLOGY

Action Against Allergy
43 The Downs
London SW20 8HG

This group offers many services aimed at bringing clinical ecology to a wider range of people. They can give information by letter or telephone, and can lend out books to members.

National Society of Research into Allergy
PO Box 45
Hinkley
Leicester LE10 1JY
Tel: 0455 635212

This organisation has helped to set up self-help groups around the country. They have produced a booklet on elimination diets. They can offer advice if you wish to set up a local group.

Society for Environmental Therapy
(Present Secretary is Mrs H. Davidson
521 Foxhall Road
Ipswich
Suffolk IP3 8LW
Tel: 0473 723552)

This is a scientific Society whose aim is to investigate illnesses caused by food, air and water. Membership is open to anyone, and there is a newsletter that will inform you of any advances in this area.

There are also a number of local self-help groups around the country. In particular, there are groups in Oxford, Cambridge, Basingstoke, St. Albans, Hythe, Seaford and Chichester. The addresses for these can be found in John Mansfield's book *The Migraine Revolution*. The National Society of Research into Allergy also has details of local groups.

ASSERTIVENESS

Redwood Women's Training Association
83 Fordwych Road
London NW2
Tel: 01-452 9261

This organisation can supply details of assertiveness courses that take place around the country.

Useful Addresses

CHIROPRACTIC

The British Chiropractors' Association
5 First Avenue
Chelmsford
Essex CM1 1RX
Tel: 0245 355487

The first of these organisations can offer a list of approved practitioners; the second can forward a list of people trained in McTimoney Chiropractic, a particularly gentle form.

The Institute of Pure Chiropractic
PO Box 127
Oxford OX1 1HH

HERBAL MEDICINE

The National Institute of Medical Herbalists
41 Hatherley Road
Winchester SO22 6RR

Most herbalists are lay practitioners; this organisation has a list of members who have been trained at the School of Herbal Medicine in Tunbridge Wells.

HOMEOPATHY

The British Homeopathic Association
27a Devonshire Street
London W1
Tel: 01-935 2163

This organisation offers a Register of Practitioners, including 350 who are also medically qualified.

The following is a list of facilities for homeopathic treatment available on the National Health Service:

The Faculty of Homeopathy
The Royal London
Homeopathic Hospital
Great Ormond Street
London WC1N 3HR
Tel: 01-837 3091

Bristol Homeopathic Hospital
Cotham
Bristol 6
Tel: 0272 731231

The Livingston Clinic: Department of Homeopathic Medicine
1 Myrtle Street
Liverpool L7 7DE
Tel: 051-709 5475

Glasgow Homeopathic Hospital
1000 Great Western Road
Glasgow G12
Tel: 041-339 0382

HYPNOTHERAPY

British Hypnotherapy Association
67 Upper Berkeley Street
London W1
Tel: 01-723 4443

The Institute of Curative Hypnotherapists
49-51 London Road
Waterlooville
Hants PO7 7EX
Tel: 0705 250123

British Society of Medical and Dental Hypnosis
42 Links Road
Ashtead
Surrey KT21 2HJ

The last of these recommends only hypnotherapists who are also medically qualified.

Useful Addresses

MIGRAINE

British Migrane Association
178a High Road
Byfleet
Weybridge
Surrey KT14 7ED
Tel: 09323 52468

The Migraine Trust
45 Great Ormond Street
London WC1N 3HD
Tel: 01-278 2676

The first of these organisations is primarily for sufferers, and aims to encourage research into migraine, to pass on information and latest findings about the problem, and to provide informal support for sufferers. They produce a newsletter three times a year. Although they do not organise local meetings, they do encourage people to meet fellow-sufferers. The Migraine Trust is more concerned with research into migraine.

There are also a number of specialist **migraine clinics** that are run throughout the country. Here you will find expert medical help for your problem, and some clinics also use relaxation and alternative approaches. You can get the address of your nearest clinic from your doctor or from the British Migraine Association's newsletter. Either way, your doctor will have to arrange an appointment on your behalf.

OSTEOPATHY

General Council and Register of Osteopaths
21 Suffolk Street
London SW1Y 4HG
Tel: 01-839 2060/930 3889

British Naturopathic and Osteopathic Association
6 Wetherall gardens
London NW3 5RR
Tel: 01-435 8728

These two organisations together represent most British osteopaths. They both keep a register of 'approved' practitioners and their addresses. They are due to be merged soon.

The British School of Osteopathy
1-4 Suffolk Street
London SW1Y 4HG
Tel: 01-930 9254

The clinic at this school treats 50,000 people a year, for modest fees.

RELAXATION

Relaxation For Living
Dunesk
29 Burwood Park Road
Walton-on-Thames
Surrey KT12 5LH
Tel: 0932 227826

This is a registered charity whose aim is to raise public awareness about the importance of true relaxation, and to set up relaxation groups around the country. Contact them for the address of your nearest group. Otherwise, it is possible to learn relaxation techniques through a correspondence course. Relaxation For Living trains volunteers to teach relaxation skills so that they can run local groups; if you are interested then contact them. They also produce numerous leaflets and booklets on relaxation.

Further Reading

HEADACHES

Migraines and Headaches   Richard Petty
(A useful book if you are   (Unwin, 1987)
particularly interested in
'alternative' approaches to
treating headaches:
acupuncture, homeopathy,
nutrition, hypnosis, and so
on.)

The Migraine Revolution   John Mansfield
(An excellent book on clinical (Thorsons, 1986)
ecology (allergies) and
headaches, although you may
find some of it rather
complex.)

Migraine   Oliver Sachs
(A good, readable   (Faber and Faber, 1970)
introduction to the topic, if a
little dated now.)

RELAXATION

Stress and Relaxation   Jane Madders
(An excellent book that is   (Martin Dunitz, 1979)
recommended by Relaxation
For Living; this charity also
produces two relaxation audio
cassettes by Jane Madders,
one of which is designed for
use with her book, and the
other for use with children.)

LIFESTYLE

Anxiety
Self Help for Your Nerves — Claire Weekes
Peace From Nervous Suffering — (Angus and Robertson)
More Help for Your Nerves
(Three excellent self-help books for anxiety problems.)

Depression
Depression – The Way Out of Your Prison — Dorothy Rowe (Routledge and Kegan Paul, 1985)
(A wise and sensitive book to help people understand and cope with their depression.)

Dealing with Depression — Kathy Nairne and Gerrilyn Smith (Women's Press, 1984)
(A valuable book specifically for women who suffer from depression. Many women share their experiences of depression in the book, and the authors offer insight and practical guidance on dealing with the problem.)

Coping with Depression — Ivy M. Blackburn (W & R Chambers, 1987)
(Also in this series)

Sleep
Insomnia — Peter Tyrer (Sheldon Press, 1978)
(A simple and readable account of sleeping problems and how best to deal with them.)

Further Reading

ASSERTION

A Woman in Your Own Right   Anne Dickson
(An important book for   (Quartet Books, 1982)
women who do not feel in
control of their own lives.
Parts of it are also highly
relevant for many men, so
don't be put off by the title if
you are male. It gives
practical advice on how to
communicate your own needs
and wishes, and how not to be
ruled by fears of criticism or
rejection.

CLINICAL ECOLOGY or FOOD ALLERGIES

Not all in the Mind   Richard Mackarness
(The classic popular book on   (Pan, 1976)
food allergies in general. If
you are interested in this
topic, Dr. Mackarness has also
written *Chemical Victims*,
published by the same
company in 1980. This deals
with sensitivities to chemicals
such as food additives.
However, if you are only
interested in the effects of
allergies on headaches, Dr
Mansfield's book (listed
above) may be more relevant
to you.)

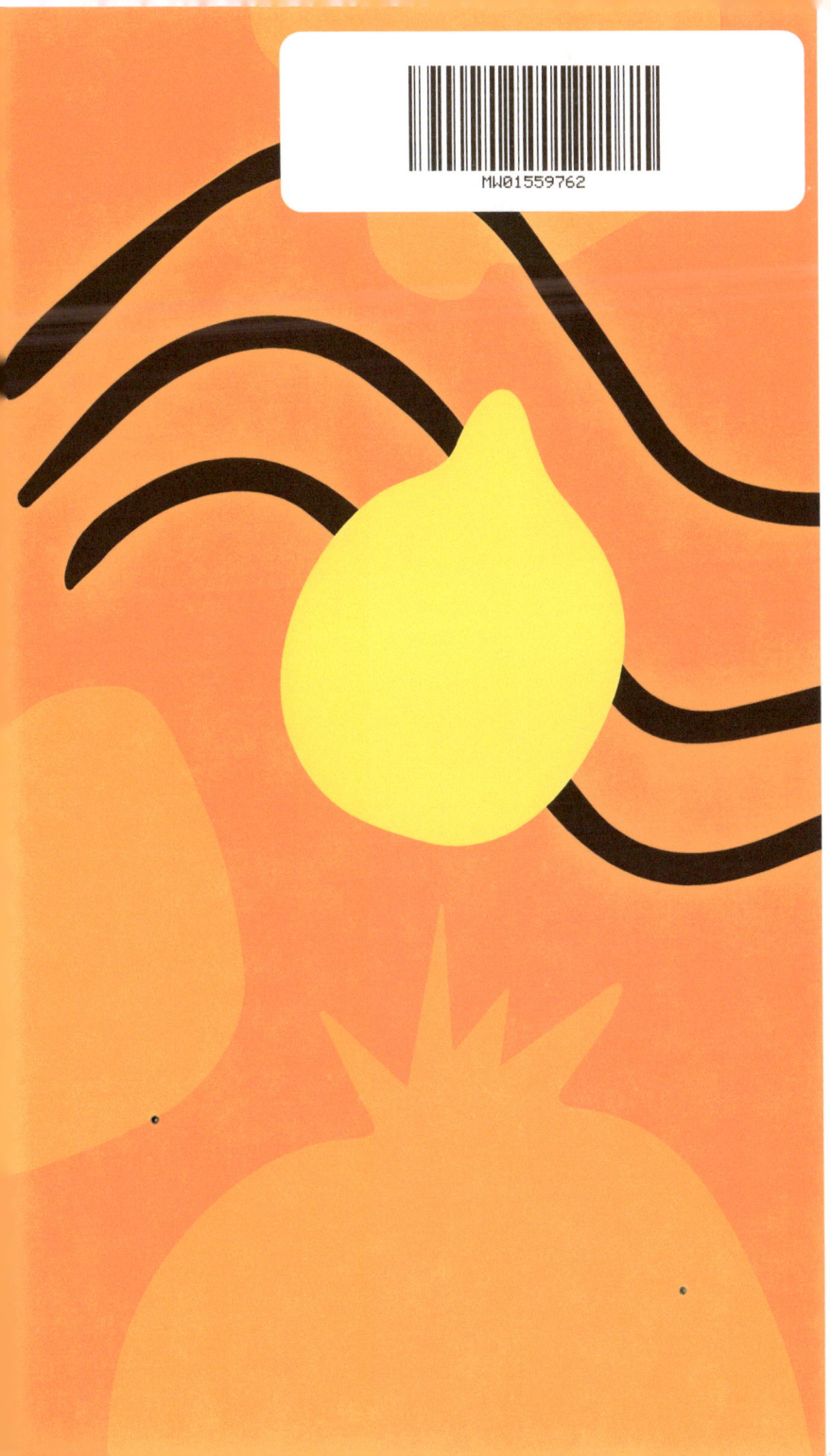

I dedicate this book to the Flourish Sisterhood.

You ladies have stood through many battles and lived to see God's blessings through various seasons of life.

You daughters of the King display how partnering with God is proof that all of our stories can be redeemed.

Self-Control: The Willing Vessel of the Lord
Copyright © 2024 by Amber Joy Thaxton
ISBN: 979-8-3304-6931-4

English Standard Version Bible. (n.d.). Bible. ESV, DailyVerses.net. Retrieved April 6, 2023, from https://dailyverses.net/

New International Version Bible. (n.d.). Bible. NIV, DailyVerses.net. Retrieved April 6, 2023, from https://dailyverses.net/

New Living Translation Bible. (n.d.). Bible. NLV, DailyVerses.net. Retrieved April 6, 2023, from https://dailyverses.net/

All rights reserved. Printed in the United States of America. No part of this book may be used or reproduced in one's business, organization, or lectures without the written permission, except for quotes or referring and giving credit to the author.

FRUITY JOURNALS

Self-control

The Willing Vessel of the Lord

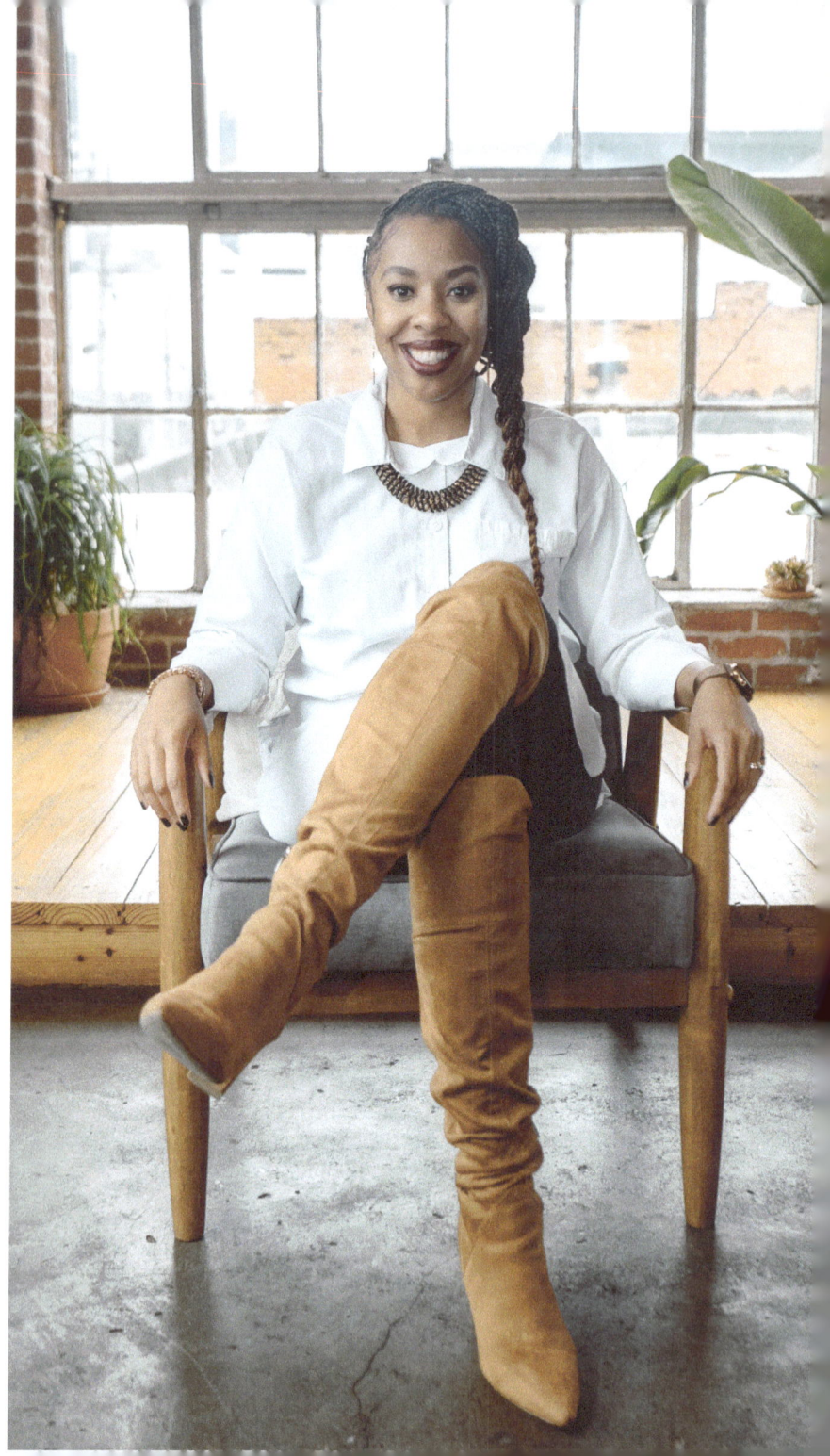

from the author

I am delighted that you have accepted the mission to be fruitful and multiply! Fruity Journals is a book series based on cultivating the fruit of God's Spirit in your life. In this journal, I share God inspired wisdom and life experiences that have pushed me closer to Him.

Fruity Journals will help the garden of your heart to flourish with peace, joy, kindness, gentleness, patience, faithfulness, self control, love and goodness. And God's word tells us that out of the abundance of the heart, the mouth speaks. You will witness God's fruit develop in your character, mind, and heart as this book takes you into the caverns of your life and offers you practical prompts for digging and soul searching.

This journal is for women just like you. Women who want to take their relationship deeper with God. Sometimes you have to go down before you can go up! Everyone likes to look at a pretty garden, but the truth is, it is messy. It is a process and every stage is not cute, but the results of health and beauty are to be treasured.

Sometimes, our gardens are nurtured by storms. The next time you go through one of life's storms, you can have the supernatural peace that keeps your mind and heart at ease. This journal series offers you daily tools to brighten your inner light and color your life with the vibrancy of God's goodness.

Okay, that is enough from me. This is the start of your spiritual self care journey.

AMBER JOY THAXTON, LPC

Yet you, Lord, are our Father. We are the clay, you are the potter; we are all the work of your hand.

Isaiah 64:8 NIV

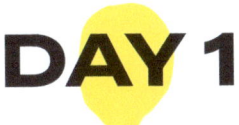
DAY 1

We all live in bodies that have sinful desires that tempt us to act out of emotion, selfishness, and pride. However, with the help of the Holy Spirit, you can experience self-control. Your spirit must become the leader of your body and soul. This happens when you realize that you are more of a spirit than you are a body, and your relationship with God is a spiritual one. As you grow in your knowledge and understanding of your Father in heaven, your spirit holds the consciousness of God.

Over the next 30 days, join me on this journey of cultivating self-control, where we will practice putting our lives on the potter's wheel for the Word of God to make and mold us into willing vessels to display His glory.

1. When you hear the word "self-control," what comes to mind for you?
2. How do you feel about your self-control today?

Self-control

DAY 1

DATE: / /   S M T W T F S

⁶For this reason I remind you to fan into flame the gift of God, which is in you through the laying on of my hands. ⁷For the Spirit that God gave us doesn't make us timid, but gives us power, love and **self-discipline.**

2 Timothy 1:6-7 NIV

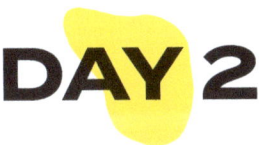

DAY 2

What gifts has God given you? What intuition seems to come naturally? How have you nurtured the gift that God has given you? Our gifts are like tiny flames that, when placed with the right elements, can become ablaze. I thought it was interesting that Paul said to fan the flame. Wind on an open flame can snuff a fire out. Wind on an open flame has the power to ravage and destroy. However, wind on a flame that is within the proper elements can be both useful and powerful.

Self-control is the empowerment of the Spirit brought on by submission. Throughout this month, we will journey through the process to become a willing vessel for the mighty, surging power of God to flow in and through our lives.

When we experience timidity, it is often because we feel out of control in some way, and so we shrink to cope. We become small in our own eyes. This passage is telling us that we have to choose to either be small and powerless or be a powerhouse of love built for the glory of God. I believe intimidation from the enemy is nothing more than a gust of wind sent to fan your flame. Consider the challenges you are facing today and envision yourself with victory! That situation you are in may just be the resistance your gifts need to rise to the occasion. You have been given everything you need to live a godly life. A godly life is a life of victory.

1. What are some of your God-given gifts?
2. How have you witnessed these gifts show up?
3. Now, consider how you can exercise and grow in them.

Self-control DAY 2

Self-control is the **empowerment** of the Holy Spirit brought on by **submission**.

DATE: / /   S M T W T F S

Like a city whose walls are broken through is a person who lacks **self-control.**

Proverbs 25:28 NIV

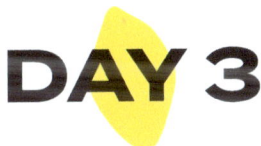

DAY 3

If you grew up in the United States like myself, it is very likely that you live in a city without walls. We can move from city to city and state to state without even noticing. What a wonderful freedom it is to travel and experience various places without inhibitors. Now, this may work well for travelers with good intentions, but what about when someone's intention is to steal, hurt, or cause destruction? The same freedom that was a privilege to one person can be misused as a path to terror for another.

When we dedicate our heart and life to God and submit ourselves to Him, we begin to experience the boundaries of love and protection that come from the Lord who reigns. God draws us in and places us in the refuge of His kingdom. As we walk with God, we learn how to share the love that was freely given to us with others. We begin to trade our selfish inhibitions for generosity and forgiveness and become fruitful citizens of God's kingdom. There is only one way to guard your heart from the pollution of the enemy, and that is to make God your refuge. God is our fortress and our shield in times of trouble. You protect the things you love, and God treasures you.

1. What are some of the ways that you have experienced God as a refuge?
2. Are there some parts of your life that need godly boundaries?

Self-control

DAY 3

DATE: / /   S M T W T F S

¹⁹The acts of the flesh are obvious: sexual immorality, impurity and debauchery; ²⁰idolatry and witchcraft; hatred, discord, jealousy, fits of rage, selfish ambition, dissensions, factions ²¹and envy; drunkenness, orgies, and the like. I warn you, as I did before, that those who live like this will not inherit the kingdom of God.

Romans 8:26 NIV

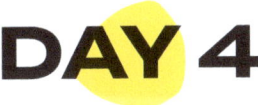

Galatians 5 provides two distinct and very different lifestyles: a life that feasts on a godly diet versus a life that becomes inebriated by selfish, worldly ambitions. The Bible gives us warning signs to help us determine which forces we are nurturing in our lives. The Bible also says that the acts of the flesh are obvious, so these are the big red flags that flap in the wind when we are faced with conflict, and our humanity is stronger than our spirit.

Take a glance at the acts of the flesh and underline any that you may have experienced in your lifetime. Now, circle any that you currently struggle with. If you keep reading through this chapter, you will come to know that verse 24 waves the winning banner because it reminds us who belong to Christ that our flesh has been crucified; it died with Christ on the Cross. The good news is, when Christ defeated the grave, the power of our flesh was also conquered. So now we live with Christ. Only the Spirit of God holds power over our mortal bodies' evil desires. You strengthen your spirit man by feeding it with daily devotion to God through praise and worship. Feast on the word of God through the reading of scripture, which renews your mind and spirit every day. It is God who gives us the power to live a faithful and fruitful life.

Write out your declaration today. Start it out by writing:
Christ has given me power over _____.

Fill in the blank with whatever struggle or temptation(s) you may find yourself struggling with.

Self-control

DATE: / /   S M T W T F S

²⁰And behold, a woman who had suffered from a discharge of blood for twelve years came up behind him and touched the fringe of his garment, ²¹for she said to herself, "If I only touch his garment, I will be made well." ²²Jesus turned, and seeing her he said, "Take heart, daughter; your faith has made you well." And instantly the woman was made well.

Psalm 32:5-7 NIV

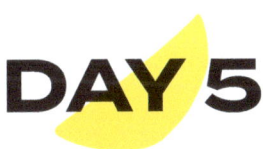

DAY 5

What a powerful demonstration of self-control by the woman with the issue of blood! This woman had chronic health issues, with one of the known symptoms being blood loss. Imagine the energy level of someone who has lost the amount of blood this woman had. Imagine how her clothes may have reeked due to the constant discharge of blood. Think about the shame she may have felt because of her ongoing predicament. Then, as she finally makes her way to Jesus, whom she has most likely heard could heal her and turn her whole life around, walks right past her to help someone else. Consider how you would have felt. What would you have done?

The passage says she said to herself, "If I only touch his garment, I will be made well." Self-talk is the loudest voice we hear. It is the voice we hear over the chatter of others' opinions. It is easier to hear our voice than the voice of God most of the time. For these very reasons, **it is important to align our beliefs with God's identity.** This was a woman whose courage and strength came from within to believe in God.

It is during moments like this that what we have put in comes out. It is moments like this that what we have studied in our daily devotions comes to the surface. It is in times of conflict that the memory verse comes to the forefront of our minds.

1. What is your self-talk like?
2. Based on what you know about God and what you're going through, write down the truth you will stand on when things become difficult.

Self-control DAY 5

DATE: /   /   S   M   T   W   T   F   S

Align your
beliefs with
God's identity.

⁴Tremble and do not sin; when you are on your beds, search your hearts and be silent.
⁵Offer the sacrifices of the righteous and trust in the LORD.

Psalm 4:4-5 NIV

DAY 6

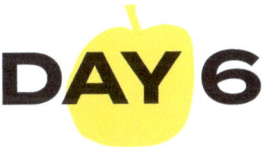

One spring vacation, we went canoeing.

It was a Monday morning and the weather was sunny. We had discussed and planned our route, but once we were in our boat, we began to notice something we could not see from the shoreline: there was a slight breeze causing the water to be choppy. As soon as we got in the water, the boat began to drift towards the forbidden sides of the bay.

I was trembling inside because I could see other big boats cutting through the ocean, causing even more waves. I noticed there were shallow areas that I was afraid to get stuck in. I began to urge my husband to row, and I was giving him directions like I had more experience than he did. We were both newbies, but the difference between me and him was that I was afraid, and it was showing. We paddled our best and still found ourselves drifting in the opposite direction. After a few minutes of fighting the waves and paddling as hard as we could, we made it back to the beach entrance.

I hopped out of the boat silently and went on a walk. I took some time to myself because I felt frustrated that my spouse did not take control and navigate us back to land with more urgency but God quickly showed me that my issue was with the wrong person. My husband is the head of our marriage, but God is the head of us both. I submitted to fear and lost sight of the holy submission to my husband and God. I was looking to my husband to be my savior, and only God can do that. In that moment, my righteous sacrifice was giving up my pride and thought process to submit to the order of the Lord. I then took a new posture, a posture of repentance and gratitude.

Has there ever been a time where you found yourself being led by fear instead of the Holy Spirit?

Self-control DAY 6

DATE: / /   S M T W T F S

⁴I also could speak like you, if you were in my place; I could make fine speeches against you and shake my head at you. ⁵But my mouth would encourage you; comfort from my lips would bring you relief.

Job 16:4-5 NIV

DAY 7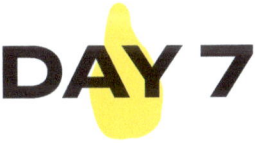

One of the places we see holy submission in the Bible is fasting. Fasting is the process of bringing our body under God's authority. While we are training our body to be led by the Spirit of God and not our natural desires, we are also directed to do so with a positive attitude and demeanor.

Why do you think it is important that we do this in secret? Our flesh often gets fed by seeking attention. Have you ever heard the saying, *'There is no such thing as bad publicity; publicity is publicity'?* Our flesh will always look for ways to be seen and glorified, but God tells us in the book of Matthew that fasting is a personal and private offering to him. It should remain discrete so that we can get the most out of it.

1. When you go through tough times, who do you usually turn to?
2. How does this passage about fasting teach you to find security in the secret place with God?

Self-control DAY 7

DATE: / /   S M T W T F S

[21] "You have heard that it was said to the people long ago, 'You shall not murder, and anyone who murders will be subject to judgment.' [22] But I tell you that anyone who is angry with a brother or sister will be subject to judgment. Again, anyone who says to a brother or sister, 'Raca,' is answerable to the court. And anyone who says, 'You fool!' will be in danger of the fire of hell. [23] "Therefore, if you are offering your gift at the altar and there remember that your brother or sister has something against you, [24] leave your gift there in front of the altar. First go and be reconciled to them; then come and offer your gift.

Matthew 5:21-24 NIV

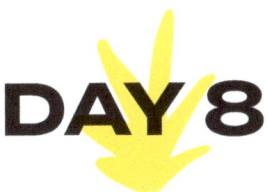

DAY 8

There are different stages to anger, and here we get a warning about how a tiny seed of anger can grow into a forest of uncontrollable fury. What most people do not know is that anger is just the tip of the iceberg. What lies underneath the surface of that feeling is really the root issue that needs to be addressed. When we feel angry, more often than not, we are feeling hurt and/or afraid.

It is difficult to control anger, which is why every part of our lives should be under holy submission. Emotions rarely stay suppressed, and this scripture references anger that goes from accusations to murder. Do not get caught up in the forest of fury because you ignored anger when it was small.

Submit your hurt and pain to the Lord and allow Him to fight your battles and heal your wounds. Remember you are healed by his stripes, and emotional wounds are included.

Self-control DAY 8

DATE: / / S M T W T F S

[23] Jesus replied, "Anyone who loves me will obey my teaching. My Father will love them, and we will come to them and make our home with them. [24] Anyone who does not love me will not obey my teaching. These words you hear are not my own; they belong to the Father who sent me.
[25] "All this I have spoken while still with you. [26] But the Advocate, the Holy Spirit, whom the Father will send in my name, will teach you all things and will remind you of everything I have said to you. [27] Peace I leave with you; my peace I give you. I do not give to you as the world gives. Do not let your hearts be troubled and do not be afraid.

Psalm 18:1-3 NIV

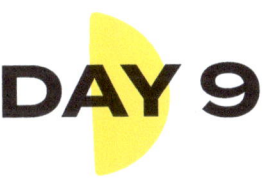

DAY 9

When my oldest child started school, I remember how much she loved her kindergarten teacher. Every day after school, she would cheerfully return home and tell us about her day. She would talk about the songs she sang, the games she played, and the things she learned in her class. It was a special excitement each day. I loved hearing about her day. From time to time, she would accidently call me by her teacher's name. "Mrs. Foster, oops, I mean mom," she would say. Did I think I was being replaced? No, of course not, but I knew she adored her and felt loved by her.

My daughter spent the majority of her day with her teacher. This is the person who would feed her, keep her safe, and make sure she was learning and having fun. And it was because of that special relationship that correction came easy with my daughter. Emery knew that when her teacher addressed an issue with her, it was coming from a place of love because her teacher built a strong bond and relationship with her.

This passage teaches us about the holy submission we are to have to God. God invested in a relationship with us through sending his son Jesus. The Son of God walked with people, prayed with them, fed them, and healed them. Jesus built relationships while on earth through words and deeds. And God, who is sovereign, knows the power of a good teacher. A good teacher does not just love the lessons; a good teacher loves the students to whom the lessons are being taught. The Holy Spirit, also referred to in the passage as the Spirit of Truth, is a gift to believers because it is evidence of God's passion for those He loves to be transformed by truth and rewarded with peace.

Read John 14:15-31 and write out the roles of the Holy Spirit. Next, write about what God is instructing you to do. Consider how you can display holy submission to God's Spirit.

Self-control DAY 9

DATE: / /   S M T W T F S

³⁰The apostles gathered around Jesus and reported to him all they had done and taught. ³¹Then, because so many people were coming and going that they did not even have a chance to eat, he said to them, "Come with me by yourselves to a quiet place and get some rest." ³²So they went away by themselves in a boat to a solitary place.

Mark 6:30-32 NIV

DAY 10

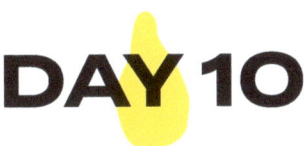

God cares about your well-being. He cares how you feel, and he is concerned about your rest. The disciples had done great work and had returned back to Jesus and shared with Him all the things that they had done and taught. How exciting it must feel for the students to tell the teacher of the great thing they did.

Jesus' response reflects how much He cares about our whole life. Many believers burn themselves out "doing things" in God's name, but here we see that God cares about our spiritual life, physical and mental. He invites his disciples to step away from the ministry of serving others and take some time to care for their own needs. There is not an area of your life that God does not care about. There is nothing too big or too small for us to bring to the Lord.

Take a moment to think about your mental, physical, and spiritual health. Are you in need of rest? Let's steal away with Jesus and plan a time to eat a good meal and simply rest.

Self-control DAY 10

God cares about your well-being.

DATE: / /   S M T W T F S

THROUGH THE POWER OF THE HOLY SPIRIT

I AM A WILLING VESSEL MADE TO DO GOOD WORK!

²¹"Besides, who would patch old clothing with new cloth? For the new patch would shrink and rip away from the old cloth, leaving an even bigger tear than before. ²²"And no one puts new wine into old wineskins. For the wine would burst the wineskins, and the wine and the skins would both be lost. New wine calls for new wineskins."

Mark 2:21-23 NLT

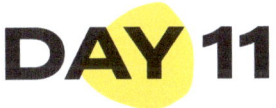

DAY 11

Religion can get old. Doing things the same old way for years, decades, and centuries can lose its meaning over time. Many of us came to know Jesus because we had an encounter with God that was like no other. Coming to know God is a process, and like any healthy relationship, it requires a level of openness to new things.

Following Jesus can feel unfamiliar and uncomfortable, and that is okay. Learning to hear God and walk by the Spirit comes with practice. Something I tell my daughter, who has a special dislike for getting things wrong, is that "practice makes better". As children of God, we do not aim to be perfect, but we must set our intention every day to be new.

Each day you wake up is a new day! Each new day needs a fresh perspective that is revitalized by the hope of Christ and the power of God that makes all things news. If you are stuck in a cycle of negative thoughts, feelings, or habits, you are experiencing human nature. When you give your life to Christ, you are given God's spirit. Just as food and water nourish your body, your spirit becomes healthier and stronger as it gains consciousness of God. Studying God's word, praying, being part of faith-based communities, and hearing testimonies are some of the ways you can feed and nourish your spirit so it becomes more alert and responsive and ultimately takes the lead over our flesh.

Consider yourself for a moment. What part of you has more influence: your flesh or your spirit? What areas of your life need to be submitted to God's will?

Self-control

DAY 11

DATE: / /   S M T W T F S

"Say to the Israelites, 'You must observe my Sabbaths. This will be a sign between me and you for the generations to come, so you may know that I am the LORD, who makes you holy.

Exodus 31:13 NIV

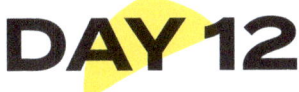

DAY 12

My husband and I are both full-time entrepreneurs with multiple businesses. I know we live in a culture where most people hear that, and they think working for yourself means that you own your time and live most of your life on vacation. While that may be a true definition for some, for many entrepreneurs, that means there is always work to be done and something constantly needs your attention. While some people are taking PTO or sleeping, you are working to make that possible for others. A successful business is one that provides a solution to a relevant problem in the world. Though we know we have been called and equipped to bring unique solutions into the world, we are also clear that we must remain submitted vessels to the will of God and not anything or anyone else.

Culture constantly encourages us to work harder, find side hustles, and grind. Every day, we are shown commercials or ads about easy ways to make money. This hustle culture dangles "the good life" like an illusive carrot, but at what expense? This toxic belief can cost you your mental wellbeing and physical health.

No matter what your career or the volunteer position you serve in, if it does not come second to your priority to obey God, it will never succeed. John 5:17 tells us that God is always at work, and when I learned that, I did not have to be. God told the Israelites in Exodus to receive rest on the Sabbath as a gift from God. Doing things differently than the world is part of what makes us different. Working a day less, tithing 10% of income or more, and fasting are all ways that God shows us that by cutting things out of our lives we are actually positioning ourselves to gain more. As we learn to will our vessels to surrender to the Spirit of God, our lives gain supernatural peace. We experience God bringing blessings into our lives that could only happen through the pruning process of obedience and self-control.

In what area of your life have you witnessed the supernatural math of less making room for more? When was the last time you rested? How are some ways you typically observe the Sabbath?

Self-control

DAY 12

DATE: / /   S M T W T F S

¹A few days later, when Jesus again entered Capernaum, the people heard that he had come home. ²They gathered in such large numbers that there was no room left, not even outside the door, and he preached the word to them. ³Some men came, bringing to him a paralyzed man, carried by four of them. ⁴Since they could not get him to Jesus because of the crowd, they made an opening in the roof above Jesus by digging through it and then lowered the mat the man was lying on. ⁵When Jesus saw their faith, he said to the paralyzed man, "Son, your sins are forgiven."

Mark 2:1-5 NIV

DAY 13

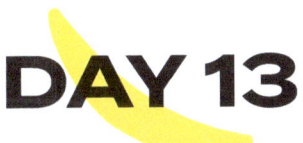

Have you ever sat with someone as they talked about what they went through and how God showed up in the mist of their trial?

I have had countless experiences when someone shared how they witnessed God show up in their life. I remember there was a time when I had no idea what to do next in my life. I had made all kinds of mistakes, and I was too ashamed to even show my face at church, because I was afraid of the judgment. I had never felt judged before, but the things the enemy tells you when you isolate yourself are distorted, and you cannot see because you are in the dark.

One day I got a knock at the door; it was my mentor. When I opened the door, I immediately felt the peace of God, and I melted into her arms. She held me as I cried and snotted all over her shoulder. God used that woman to embrace me and remind me that I am loved.

He used her to usher in His light and His truth in the midst of me feeling like a depressed failure. That day marked a turning point for me. I repented, and I leaned on my mentor for accountability as I began to seek God and walk in His grace and mercy.

Testimonies are our stories marked by our point of view of God intervening in our lives. We have to fight against the shame the enemy tries to keep us bound by to stop us from telling of our pain and shortcomings. But if we let God in, He will save us, and we will live to tell of His glory.

What's your story?
Think back to a time you witnessed God intervene in your life.
I dare you to make a plan to tell someone about it.

Self-control

DAY 13

DATE: / /   S M T W T F S

You did not choose me, but I chose you and appointed you so that you might go and bear fruit—fruit that will last—and so that whatever you ask in my name the Father will give you. This is my command: Love each other.

John 15:16-17 NIV

DAY 14

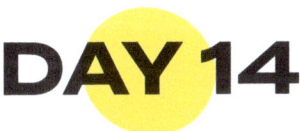

I am a recovering people-pleaser. As a little girl, I loved pleasing my parents and teachers by doing a good job. I noticed early on how hearing the words "good job" filled my bucket to the brim! Unfortunately, I carried this mindset over into my Christian faith. I often want to know that I am pleasing God, and sometimes I have moments when I get worried about whether I should or could be doing something better with my time or resources.

However, God often reminds me that I did not choose him. He chose me and put me in a position to be his hands and feet. He has well equipped those who love him and are called. He has given us autonomy over our prayer requests because this is a holy partnership. When willing vessels surrender to the mission of God to love others and continue the work of Christ, we see the reveal of a dynamic union.

Consider your unique relationship with God. In what ways have you seen your union with God bear good fruit?

Self-control

DAY 14

DATE: / /   S M T W T F S

⁵For those who live according to the flesh set their minds on the things of the flesh, but those who live according to the Spirit set their minds on the things of the Spirit. ⁶For to set the mind on the flesh is death, but to set the mind on the Spirit is life and peace. ⁷For the mind that is set on the flesh is hostile to God, for it does not submit to God's law; indeed, it cannot.

Romans 8:5-7 ESV

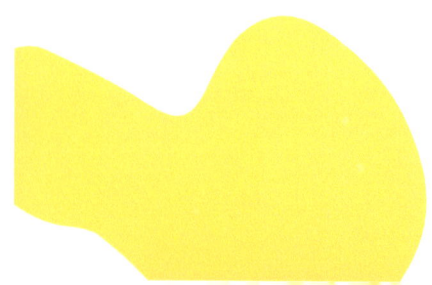

DAY 15

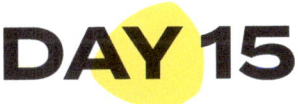

Self-control is a fruit produced by your walk with God. Our acceptance of Christ in our lives transformed everything about how we see God, ourselves, and the world. When you become a willing vessel for God's spirit, your selfish desires no longer satisfy you the way they once did. Those selfish desires are still present but no longer hold the same weight.

The spirit of God inside of us shifts our mindsets to think and meditate on God's goodness, faithfulness, and will. We now consider what God's will is for our lives. We consider what would bring God praise and glory out of any circumstance. The ecosystem of faith is amazing; this holy submission harvests even more fruit. When our minds are governed by the spirit of God, it empowers us to work out the will of God and gives us peace in the process. Hallelujah, and thank you, Jesus!

Allow me to add a disclaimer. God is a spirit, and there are going to be times that you make a misstep. Mistakes and shortcomings do not make you any less of a child of God. They do not make you any less loved by God. In fact, God has created a fail-proof system that helps to reposition us back on the path called grace. Grace is God's unmerited (unearned) favor, and the word of God says that it is sufficient in times of trouble. 2 Corinthians 12:12 says that his grace is actually made perfect in your weakness. **Remember, your weaknesses are only revealed when you make an effort.**

Today, take a moment to reread the statements about how to be led by God's spirit that are underlined. Consider God's will for your life today and journal about the effort you can put forth with the help of the Holy Spirit to work that out.

Self-control

DAY 15

DATE: / /   S M T W T F S

Your weaknesses
are only revealed
when you make
an effort.

Do not be envious of evil men, Nor desire to be with them;
For their minds plot violence,
And their lips talk of trouble [for the innocent]

Through [skillful and godly] wisdom a house [a life, a home, a family] is built,
And by understanding it is established [on a sound and good foundation],
And by knowledge its rooms are filled
With all precious and pleasant riches.

Proverbs 24:1-4 AMP

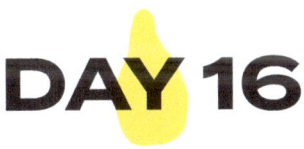

DAY 16

Some of us hear the word wicked and think of the witch with the green face and black hat from the Wizard of Oz. Although the ol girl was in need of a savior, the wicked can look just like me and you. A wicked person is someone who opposes God and is immoral. These individuals can be funny, beautiful, wealthy, smart, and intriguing, but their greatest flaw is that they believe they know better than God. Be careful who you are attracted to. God sees beyond the surface and knows the heart of every person.

A vessel of God skillfully constructs their life with wisdom through consideration of the will of God. If you desire to become more understanding of the will and ways of God, spend time in communication with God. Listen more than you speak. When you read the word of God, take time to chew on it and consider how it applies to you or how it brings context to the character and nature of God.

How would you describe how you are constructing your life? What's your process for making decisions? Is there a particular valley of decision that you are in today? Let's bring this to God in prayer and trust him as the master architect in your life.

Self-control

DAY 16

DATE: / /   S M T W T F S

²⁷So then, whoever eats the bread or drinks the cup of the Lord in an unworthy manner will be guilty of sinning against the body and blood of the Lord. ²⁸Everyone ought to examine themselves before they eat of the bread and drink from the cup. ²⁹For those who eat and drink without discerning the body of Christ eat and drink judgment on themselves.

1 Corinthians 11:27-29 NIV

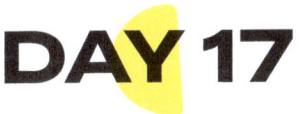

DAY 17

I remember when I first learned about the Lord's Supper as a child. I was warned to take it seriously and to examine my heart before I took part. To this day, I still feel the weight of my mother's words. When you observe the Lord's supper, it is a holy moment! It is a time like no other that we focus our attention and hearts on a love like no other.

While preparing to take the Lord's Supper, we remember with thanksgiving that Jesus gave his life as an atonement on the cross for our sins. In one moment, Jesus rights our every wrong and offers us a way to escape eternal separation from him so that we can live a new life in harmony with our creator. Harmony with God requires careful consideration every day. As believers we must increase our self-awareness. Yes, during the Lord's supper, but every day we pick up our cross, we must be careful to consider all the other things that the enemy tries to load us up with for the day as well.

Lay down the pressure to please everyone around you. Set aside the stress of trying to achieve worldly success. Let go of the fear of the future. Peel off the negative labels and lies others have tried to pin on you. You were never designed to carry these burdens. Jesus demonstrated how to carry your cross. Carry your calling to be a light and make disciples with the confidence that God has done the heaviest lifting, sent his son Jesus to pave the way, and gave you His spirit so you empower you!

Reflection time! Use these questions to consider how you are doing.

How do I feel?
What has happened to me recently?
What do I need?

Self-control

DAY 17

DATE: / /   S M T W T F S

Oh, that their hearts would be inclined to fear me and keep all my commands always, so that it might go well with them and their children forever!

Deuteronomy 5:29 NIV

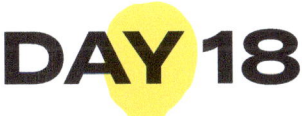

DAY 18

This was a statement made by God after Moses had delivered the 10 Commandments to the Israelites. Here, God describes an integral component of self-control that will be necessary to follow and obey his commands—an inclined heart.

Some of God's instructions are clear expectations for us and the 10 commandments are one of those. God lists 10 dos and don'ts; though they are clear, they will still require a properly postured heart. However, it is interesting that as clear as these instructions are, God still mentioned that it requires a heart that is positioned to reverence and honor him as Lord. This tells us that clear instructions are not enough for obedience. It is the direction our heart is facing when we are given instructions that ensures our success rate.

Is your heart leaning towards God? We must position ourselves to be closer to God than we are to any other desire or influence. We make a habit to carefully follow God by positioning ourselves mentally, physically, and spiritually. Walking in obedience is paying attention to the path outlined by God and His Spirit and meditation is the act of focusing our minds' eye on the things above. We weaken our flesh by strengthening our spirit. We feed our spirit with God's word, prayer, worship, gratitude, fellowship, etc. This is how we will make our vessel a pleasing sacrifice to the Lord.

Take this promise to heart today. Know that as you obey God's instructions, he promises you that you and your children's lives will all work out.

Self-control

DAY 18

DATE: / /   S M T W T F S

¹In the spring, at the time when kings go off to war, David sent Joab out with the king's men and the whole Israelite army. They destroyed the Ammonites and besieged Rabbah. But David remained in Jerusalem.
²One evening David got up from his bed and walked around on the roof of the palace. From the roof he saw a woman bathing. The woman was very beautiful, ³and David sent someone to find out about her. The man said, "She is Bathsheba, the daughter of Eliam and the wife of Uriah the Hittite."

2 Samuel 11:1-3 NIV

DAY 19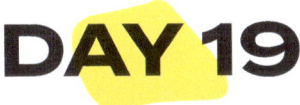

I grew up in Southern California, and one of my most distinct memories comes from high school. I can remember so vividly the lunchroom where we gathered for meals and assemblies, the front office where you'd have to go to get a late slip if you were tardy, and the echoing hallways where all the students would have to pass each day to commute to their next class. During the hours when students should be in class, there would be a security guard or hall monitor on guard. And if you were caught in the hallway after the bell rang, there would be a problem. The Hall Monitor would ask, "Where are you supposed to be?"

David, who is described famously in the Bible as a man after God's own heart, is the same person who had other struggles. Chapter 11 started by letting us know 3 important things: a) This is a time when Kings should be off to war; b) David's army was doing well; c) David remained in the comfort of his home. It was clear that David was called by God and trained his army well, but it was also clear that he had some weaknesses that got him into real trouble. Read the full chapter to see how David's lack of self-control ended up hurting himself and others.

An important key to developing self-control is being aware of both your strengths and your weaknesses. Do not put yourself under unnecessary pressure. If you have issues with overeating, do not go to a buffet. If you have an issue with drinking, avoid the bar. If you have issues overspending, do not keep applying for credit cards. We all have things that attempt to tug our hearts in the opposite direction of God.

Ask yourself today, Where am I? Am I putting myself in situations that help bring out my best? Am I putting myself in situations that get the best of me?

Self-control DAY 19

DATE: / /   S M T W T F S

Do not answer a fool according to his folly, or you yourself will be just like him.

Proverbs 26:4 NIV

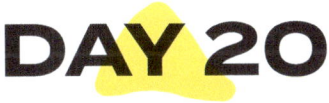
DAY 20

I have 5 siblings, and there was about a 10-year age difference between the first set of children and the last set. I am a proud middle child, and peacemaking is the name of my game. This probably has a great deal to do with why I became a Licensed Professional Therapist, but way before all the training and certifications, I found myself in my teenage years wanting to help my family reconcile. I found value in all parties being heard and feelings being validated.

Over time, I learned that not everyone wants peace. I learned that not everyone seeks wisdom and understanding, but if I was not careful, I would find myself entangled in long discussions with emotionally stunted individuals, and I found myself feeling frustrated.

Have you ever been in a conversation with someone that grew tense? Did the volume of the conversation begin to increase? Did responses get traded for comebacks, and defensiveness creates a deafness to truth?

When you find yourself in conflict and you are in a position to confront injustice, wrongdoing, or unfairness, **remember that God sees the heart.** We can communicate our thoughts and feelings and treat others with respect and dignity no matter their level of ignorance they stoop to.

Michelle Obama once said, "When they go low, we go higher."

Are you comfortable with confrontation? Confrontation has a bad reputation but it really just means to face something. What about your approach to facing challenges do you find most effective? What are the parts of confronting you find challenging?

Self-control DAY 20

God sees
your heart.

DATE: / /   S M T W T F S

YOU ARE

WE ARE

THE POTTER...

THE CLAY.

¹²For just as the body is one and has many members, and all the members of the body, though many, are one body, so it is with Christ. ¹³For in one Spirit we were all baptized into one body—Jews or Greeks, slaves[d] or free—and all were made to drink of one Spirit. ¹⁴For the body does not consist of one member but of many.

1 Corinthians 12:12-14 ESV

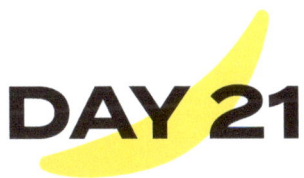

DAY 21

God created you for connection. You are unique, and what you bring to the body of Christ cannot be compared to what someone else brings. Your unique perspective, personality, and ways that you support others are solely unique to you. If nobody has told you lately, we need you. We need your wisdom. We need your knowledge. We need your mercy, faith, etc. We are all granted spiritual gifts that are designed for the building of God's kingdom, but what is a gift if never discovered?

Many of our gifts become exposed through life situations that elicit our special function. A person might be going through something challenging, and through the impression of the Holy Spirit, you share the plans God has in store for them. There is an unexpected loss, and suddenly you see an opportunity to put those culinary skills to good use to support a grieving family. You walk into a room only to notice there is something dark or unusual. You may have the ability to break down information and make complicated matters teachable.

The body of Christ is not the same without you. Fight the urges to isolate yourself or compare and minimize your amazing qualities. Will your vessel lend itself to the unification of the bride of Christ?

How do you view the body of Christ?
Where do you see yourself in it?

Self-control DAY 21

DATE: / /   S M T W T F S

God also said to Moses, "Say to the Israelites, 'The Lord,[a] the God of your fathers—the God of Abraham, the God of Isaac and the God of Jacob—has sent me to you.'
"This is my name forever, the name you shall call me from generation to generation

1 Samuel 18:14 NIV

DAY 22

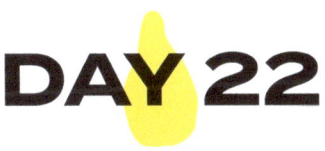

During an unforgettable encounter with God through a burning bush, Moses receives instructions to face one Pharaoh who had brutally kept him and his people enslaved. Upon receiving the instructions, Moses asks how he should refer to God to the Isrealites when he conveys the instructions of this mighty mission. God did not say Creator of the Universe; He did not say King of Kings; He said I AM who I AM. Later, He said, "The Lord and God of your fathers." God is a relational God. He loves us deeply and wants you to know him on a personal level.

In other words, God was saying I am the one who has always been there. Before the Israelites existed, God had them in mind. Abraham was over 70 years old when he promised him a nation, and his wife Sarah was barren. Maybe you're unfamiliar with I Am, but you may have heard of the God of Isaac, who trusted God enough to lay on the altar when there was no other sacrifice to offer. God was saying maybe you do not know me just yet, but take the word of your great-grandfather, grandfather, and father. These men walked with me, talked with me, and one wrestled with God! Take their word for it. There are times following God can feel uncomfortable. And trying to find the words to express what he is leading you to do can be difficult. Each day you take a step of faith to follow Christ, you are willing your vessel to surrender to God's mission.

Looking back and reflecting on moments and testimonies of those you know encountered God. I pray that this will be like a hit of lightning to our Spirit and stir your heart to follow God with boldness today.

Self-control DAY 22

DATE: / /   S M T W T F S

[28] So Jesus said to them, "When you have lifted up the Son of Man, then you will know that I am he, and that I do nothing on my own authority, but speak just as the Father taught me. [29] And he who sent me is with me. He has not left me alone, for I always do the things that are pleasing to him." [30] As he was saying these things, many believed in him.

John 8:28-30 ESV

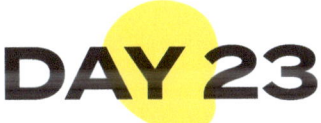
DAY 23

As we comb through scripture and learn what it really means to have self-control, we witness Jesus, our savior, display in 3D full color what it means to be a willing vessel. Jesus was in sync with God. Like a dance duet made up of two talented performers, yet one takes the lead for the movements to flow and unfold into a rhythmic ensemble. Jesus made it clear that his authority and power were given to him by God himself. Therefore, he did not seek the approval of the Pharisees to permit him to proclaim God's love, truth, and grace.

Every word spoken by Jesus is and was rooted from the foundation of God Almighty. The fruit of a believer's life is eternal and has the power to influence generations to come. Never think of yourself or your actions as small. Everything you do matters, especially what you do out of a willing heart for the building of God's kingdom.

If you are wondering how you will live the life patterned after Jesus, remember that it is not dependent on your own ability. Even Christ was taught and sent. And we have the added insurance of God's presence!

What is the passage saying to you?
In what area of your life do you need God's guidance?

Self-control **DAY 23**

DATE: / /   S M T W T F S

The Lord is not slow in keeping his promise, as some understand slowness. Instead he is patient with you, not wanting anyone to perish, but everyone to come to repentance.

2 Peter 3:9 NIV

DAY 24

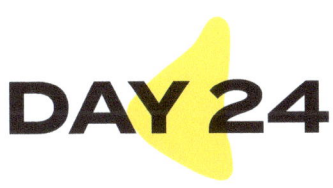

God knows you so well. He knows that it takes time for us to learn of his love. It takes time for us to accept and adjust to true love. Most of us have lived with counterfeit versions of love for so long. Maybe you were always told you were loved but did not always see corresponding actions, or maybe you grew up in a home where affection was not displayed and having a roof over your head and your basic needs provided for were supposed to be enough. No matter how you grew up, people over time will disappoint you. I am not saying that to be a Debbie Downer; it is just a fact. I have disappointed people; you have also disappointed people, whether intended or not. This is one of the very reasons we need God, because without him we can do nothing.

This passage tells us so much about God's character. It shows us that we serve a God who is gentle and patient in nature. Oftentimes we want the fast track to success, the magic pill for weight loss, or the knight in shining armor, but God's approach to our growth is an endearing one. He loves us so deeply and desires for us to live in eternity with him. He patiently works with us and takes time molding us into vessels for good use. He does not crush us, pressure us, or smother us. He guides us with truth and surrounds us with his love as he offers us new life. Repentance is the act of acknowledging your sin and turning away from death and towards life.

Take a moment to examine your life and heart and ask the Holy Spirit to show you if there are any areas in your life that need repentance. Pray for the lost and those who may feel far from God that they may turn back towards God and experience revival.

Self-control DAY 24

DATE: / /   S M T W T F S

[10] Then the word of the Lord came to Samuel: [11] "I regret that I have made Saul king, because he has turned away from me and has not carried out my instructions." Samuel was angry, and he cried out to the Lord all that night.

1 Samuel 15:10-11 NIV

DAY 25

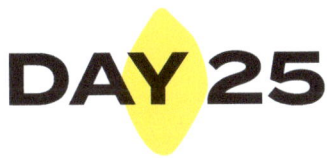

Saul was chosen by God himself to be king over Israel. God sent Saul the support he needed to be successful even when Saul did not see himself as capable or qualified. The prophet Samuel was one of many that God sent into Saul's life to help support and guide him. God sent specific instructions for Saul and his army to attack the Amalekities and totally destroy them. The Amalekities came against Israel as they were fleeing from Egypt, and God was carrying out judgment on a nation that came up against His people. (May this be a reminder that God has your back.)

Saul partially obeys by attacking the Amalekites but does not complete the mission by choosing to spare King Agag and keep some of the livestock. Saul struggled with self-control. Somewhere along his life, his heart shifted from a humble position to one that was haughty. Saul made the decision to do things his way because his way was more beneficial. Proverbs 14:12 reads, There is a way which seemeth right unto a man, but the end thereof are the ways of death.

It is not enough to be a partially willing vessel of the Lord. To follow God, you have to walk by faith, more than you do logic. Logic is limited. Logic requires you to fully comprehend what to do and how to do it, but self-control is a fruit that comes from a relationship with the Spirit of God, which operates in another realm. Our earthly knowledge could not truly begin to explain the origins of who God is and the scope of his mission. The key to self-control is knowing that God loves you and has the best for you in mind. To be a willing vessel of the Lord requires us to trust him more than we understand Him.

Read 1 Samuel Chapter 15. What does this reading tell you about God's character and the importance of self-control?

Self-control **DAY 25**

DATE: / /   S M T W T F S

The Lord lives! Praise be to my Rock!
 Exalted be God my Savior!
He is the God who avenges me,
 who subdues nations under me,
 who saves me from my enemies.
You exalted me above my foes;
 from a violent man you rescued me.
Therefore I will praise you, Lord, among the nations;
 I will sing the praises of your name.

Psalm 18:46-49 NIV

DAY 26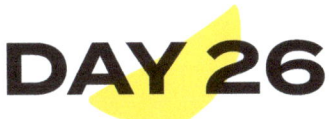

There is something powerful about reflecting on your life and reminiscing on all that God has brought you through. Self-control can be one of the toughest fruits to see blossom in our lives because there are so many things that attempt to influence and control us. Money, fear, comparison—so many things attempt to rule over our hearts and existence.

David wrote this song after God delivered him from Saul and his enemies. He was wanted dead, and many people turned on him out of fear of what would happen if they helped him even though they knew he was innocent. How overwhelming it must have felt to be betrayed by those who once said they loved you and were your friends, but David knew a love that was without condition.

It took self-control to will his vessel to trust God when he was hiding in caves and running for his life. Meanwhile, God was avenging him and making ways out of no way. David sang praises, worshiped God, and exalted Him. I know what it is like to struggle with health. I have felt the pit in my stomach that hit after swiping my card for groceries, only to hear the piercing beep that signals "insufficient funds." My flesh wanted to cry out and complain that I was forgotten by God, but lifting my eyes towards the heavens and worshiping God when things did not look great was the only path forward out of the dark pit I felt my mind and heart slipping into.

To walk by faith is to live with a spiritual awareness that God is on the throne and always at work. What are you experiencing currently that feels like it is trying to rule over you? I invite you to take a moment to praise God and lift up the name of Jesus. Worship wages war on the enemy.

Self-control DAY 26

DATE: / /   S M T W T F S

⁵In the same way, you who are younger, submit yourselves to your elders. All of you, clothe yourselves with humility toward one another, because,

"God opposes the proud
    but shows favor to the humble."

⁶Humble yourselves, therefore, under God's mighty hand, that he may lift you up in due time. ⁷Cast all your anxiety on him because he cares for you.

1 Peter 5:5-7 NIV

DAY 27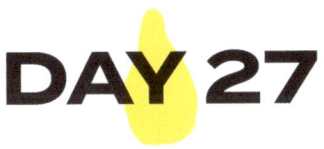

We all encounter storms from time to time. I have a courageous friend who enjoys going outside when the sky begins to look funny and the wind picks up. Chasing storms is intriguing to her! I love my friend, and with that said, we could not be more different.

Storms usually signal danger to me.
Once, in the middle of the night, we had a really big storm in Tulsa, Oklahoma, and when I was awakened by tornado sirens, I dizzily stumbled to the bathroom and got oriented to what was taking place. This night, I had a different response.

Usually, I gather my little ones and cower into a closet as I hope for God to protect us. This time was different. See what the wind and rain did not know, was that I had been in a spiritual storm leading up to this moment, and in the light of those events I had been exercising my heavenly prayer language. I had been taking captive any thoughts of fear and dread in my mind.

The Spirit of God in me had been stirred, and I was in touch with the power God had given me through Christ! I walked over to the window, and spoke to the storm. I prayed with a boldness. My friend may chase storms, but with the help of the Holy Spirit, I faced the storm, and it stopped within minutes!

Each moment we live is an opportunity to trust God and walk by faith. I encourage you, if you have not already, to ask God to fill you with His Spirit. If you have received God's spirit, now is the time to stir your faith with prayer and awaken your spirit today! Jesus left us with someone greater—the Holy Spirit is your helper and guide. Face your storm today, and with all the power God has given you, rebuke it!

Self-control

DAY 27

DATE: / / S M T W T F S

¹As he went along, he saw a man blind from birth. ²His disciples asked him, "Rabbi, who sinned, this man or his parents, that he was born blind?"

³"Neither this man nor his parents sinned," said Jesus, "but this happened so that the works of God might be displayed in him. ⁴As long as it is day, we must do the works of him who sent me. Night is coming, when no one can work. ⁵While I am in the world, I am the light of the world.

John 9:1-5 NIV

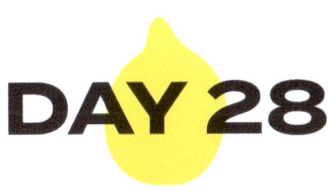

DAY 28

Have you ever asked yourself, "Why me?" Why did I have to grow up in this circumstance?" "What did I do to deserve this treatment?" "Why do I not have (fill in the blank)?" Life has many mysteries, but God's ability to use them for his glory is certain. Very often, we spend so much time trying to find out why or how we got into certain situations, but there comes a time when surrendering it to the Lord becomes necessary.

The man in this passage was born blind, and the disciples were seeking to understand who was at fault, the man or his parents. However, Jesus redirects their attention from who should be at fault to who should be glorified. I remember the moment that I received an unfavorable report from my doctor after there was a lump discovered in my breast. I was sent to see a specialist for further testing. I remember the pit I felt in my stomach and all the "what if" scenarios that all lead to the same bleak ending. I began to think about how I never met my grandmother because she died so early. My mind became bombarded by thoughts of my aunts on my mother's side who had also passed away from health issues and tragic circumstances.

I remember the self-control that was required to take captive every thought that raised itself up against the word of God. I believed in my heart that I was healed by his stripes, but my mind was another battle. Each day leading up to the next appointment, I reminded my mind of what my heart believed. I walked into that appointment holding on to the belief that Jesus' work on the cross was enough, and I came out of the appointment knowing the blood of Jesus covers sin and genetics. I know God did a miracle for me. I share this because I know life is no cakewalk, and I believe that, like that blind man, God also wants to use my story and your story to display his wonderful power.

Can you remember a time in your life where you witnessed God turn a situation around?

Self-control DAY 28

DATE: / /   S M T W T F S

Keep my commands and you will live; guard my teachings as the apple of your eye. Bind them on your fingers; write them on the tablet of your heart. Say to wisdom, "You are my sister," and to insight, "You are my relative."

Proverbs 7:2-4 NIV

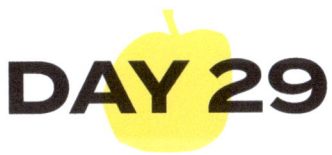

DAY 29

How do you keep a command you do not know? It can be tempting to do what feels right, but the Bible says in Proverbs 14:12 that there is a way that seems right to a man, but it ends in death. Our emotions are not meant to be in the driving seat of our lives. It can be tempting to be led by what feels "right." Our emotions are like magnifying glasses that illuminate what is happening within us. Even our ideas must be examined and measured by our true beliefs and values.

Your beliefs are established by what you place your trust in and invest your time to understand. Do you believe that God can be trusted? Trusting God is the only way you will ever truly be able to accept the truth and follow his directions. Following God's commands is the way to life.

Quality time is one of my top love languages because the time I spend offering undivided attention to my loved ones leads to greater intimacy and deeper love. I learn more about their unique qualities. There is space to be curious and ask questions. There is no substitute for quality time with God. Wisdom comes from above, and the insight you need to live a wonderful and godly life comes from the Spirit of God.

Though God is with you all the time, how do you make the most of the time? How do you hear and experience God?

Self-control DAY 29

DATE: / /   S M T W T F S

Those of us who are strong and able in the faith need to step in and lend a hand to those who falter, and not just do what is most convenient for us. Strength is for service, not status. Each one of us needs to look after the good of the people around us, asking ourselves, "How can I help?"

Romans 15:1-2 MSG

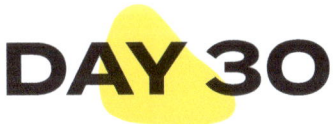

DAY 30

Followers of Christ are to lead with love and kindness. The Holy Spirit teaches us how to be gentle and meet others where they are. Oftentimes, as believers, we grow in our faith and understanding of God over time, but when we see someone else struggling or having a setback, we can become impatient with them and try to pressure others to change or get it together quickly.

The journey that has matured your faith was unique. There is no blueprint for heart change; there is only the supernatural work of God that is able to bring each of us to repentance.

If there is someone in your life that you know God has better for, be gentle in your approach. Consider how prayer, encouragement, and gentle words can make a difference.

Self-control

DAY 30

DATE: / / / /   S M T W T F S

My heart is good soil.

Each day with the help of the Holy Spirit, I survey my heart.

I believe when I confess my sins, I am forgiven.

I believe when I cast my cares, I am free.

Day after day, God replenishes me from His well of living water.

And as a result, my life is blossoming with Godly fruit.

Amen.

NOTES

DATE: / / S M T W T F S

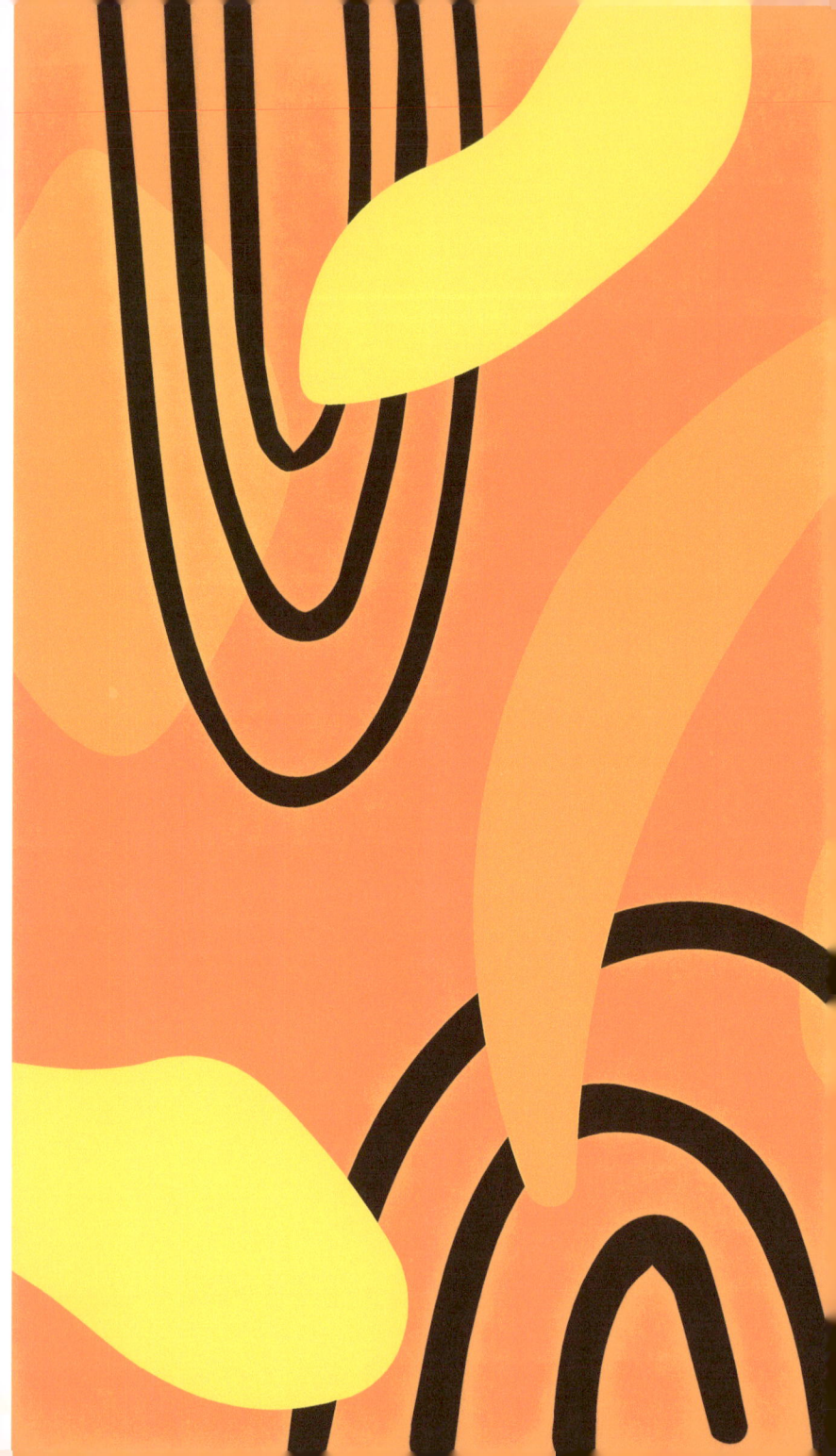

Printed in the USA
CPSIA information can be obtained
at www.ICGtesting.com
JSHW041938211024
72114JS00002B/3